the **Voice**
___

Heman-Ackah
Sataloff
Hawkshaw

the Voice: A Medical Guide for Achieving and Maintaining a Healthy Voice

ISBN 978-0-9758862-4-3

Notice: With ongoing research and improvements in technology, the information and applications discussed in this text are constantly changing and are subject to the practitioner's professional judgment and interpretation in accordance to the clinical situation. Readers are advised to check the most current information provided by the manufacturers of drugs and technologies to verify the recommended usage and/or dose, method and duration of administration, and contraindications. Neither the authors nor publisher assume any liability for injury or damage arising from use of the information in this publication.

Photographs: Cover photos courtesy of M. Peters, University Singers, John J. Cali School of Music, Montclair State University, Upper Montclair, NJ. Inset photos courtesy of R. Sataloff, Y. Heman-Ackah, and iStockPhoto.com (claudiaveja, sturti). All photographs appearing on the covers of this text are intended to portray only artistic performance or an occupation, and their use does not imply or represent the presence of any medical condition in these persons.

Library of Congress Cataloging-in-Publication data [in preparation]

The Voice: A Medical Guide for Achieving and Maintaining a Healthy Voice
by Yolanda D. Heman-Ackah, Robert T. Sataloff, and Mary J. Hawkshaw.
p.; cm.
includes bibliographic references and index.
ISBN 978-0-9758862-4-3.
1.

© 2013 Science & Medicine, Inc.
All rights reserved. Printed in USA.

This title is also available as an e-book at **www.sciandmed.com/**.

No part of this publication may be reproduced, copied, reprinted, or transmitted in any form by any means, electronic or mechanical, including photocopy, recording, website, or information storage and retrieval system, without the prior written permission of the publisher.

Permission for photocopying material in this volume or for use in academic course-packets, electronic or print, may be obtained through the Copyright Clearance Center, 222 Rosewood Drive, Danvers MA 01923, USA, www.CopyRight.com.

Science & Medicine
PO Box 313
Narberth, PA 19072

www.sciandmed.com
800-888-0028 / 610-660-8097
fax 610-660-0348

the *Voice*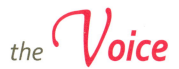

A Medical Guide for Achieving and Maintaining a Healthy Voice

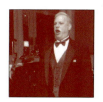

Yolanda D. Heman-Ackah, MD
Robert T. Sataloff, MD, DMA
Mary J. Hawkshaw, RN, BSN, CORLN

SCIENCE & MEDICINE

iv   *the Voice*

Contents

	Introduction	... vi
	About the Authors	... viii
1	Anatomy: Where is the Voice Produced?	... 1
2	How is the Voice Produced?	... 15
3	How do I Maintain Longevity of my Voice?	... 27
4	How do I Find a Voice Doctor and Voice Care Team?	... 37
5	When Should I See a Voice Doctor?	... 51
6	What can I Expect During a Visit to a Voice Doctor?	... 59
7	What are the Possible Causes of Voice Problems?	... 77
8	What is Reflux and How does it Contribute to Voice Problems?	... 103
9	What does it Mean to Have a "Weak" Vocal Fold?	... 119
10	What are Options for Non-Surgical Treatment of Voice Problems?	... 129
11	When is Voice Surgery Indicated?	... 135
	Index	... 151

▲ Dedication

To our patients and our students.

▲ Introduction

This book is meant to be an informational source for professional voice users on how to care for and maintain the longevity of the voice from a purely medical perspective. This is not a book on vocal pedagogy, but rather a guide to common medical problems that can affect the voice and to common vocal difficulties that can develop from ineffective voice use. This book also serves as a resource guide for finding and recognizing appropriate voice care.

This book is purposely designed to be easy to read and is intended for non-medical voice professionals. Singing teachers, those studying vocal performance and acting, acting voice teachers, and voice coaches may find this material particularly useful. However, the material within this book applies to all voice professionals, including singers, actors, lawyers, public speakers, politicians, teachers, phone operators, stock brokers, salesmen, corporate executives, and others who use their voice in their profession.

To our knowledge, this is the first book on the medical aspects of the voice and vocal health written by physicians for voice professionals.

YDH
RTS
MJH

▲ About the Authors

YOLANDA D. HEMAN-ACKAH, MD, FACS

Yolanda D. Heman-Ackah, MD, is a laryngologist who specializes in professional voice care. She is board certified by the American Board of Otolaryngology and is a fellow of the American Academy of Otolaryngology–Head and Neck Surgery. She received her Bachelor of Arts degree in Psychology and her Doctor of Medicine degree from Northwestern University as part of the Honors Program in Medical Education. Following her residency in otolaryngology–head and neck surgery at the University of Minnesota, she completed a fellowship in professional voice care and laryngology under the preceptorship of Robert T. Sataloff, MD, DMA at the American Institute for Voice and Ear Research and Jefferson Medical College of Thomas Jefferson University in Philadelphia, PA. In addition to her medical training, Dr. Heman-Ackah is also a professionally trained dancer, a musician, and a vocalist.

She founded and directed the Voice Center at the University of Illinois at Chicago upon completion of her fellowship. After a few years in Chicago, she joined the practice of Dr. Robert T. Sataloff in Philadelphia, PA. After almost 10 years in practice with Dr. Sataloff, she was recruited by the Cleveland Clinic to head the Section of Laryngology and direct the Voice Center at the Cleveland Clinic. After returning to Philadelphia, she is currently Director and owner of the Philadelphia Voice Center, which specializes in profesional voice care and other aspects of otolaryngology–head and neck surgery as they pertain to the performing artist and professional voice user. She is an active member of the academic faculties of Drexel University College of Medicine, where she currently holds the position of Associate Professor, and Thomas Jefferson University, where she is adjunct Associate Professor. She is the National Medical Advisor for the Voice and Speech Trainer's Association (VASTA) and is actively involved in VASTA, the Voice Foundation, the National Association of Teachers of Singing (NATS), the Latin Academy of Recording Arts and Sciences, and the National Academy of Recording Arts and Sciences (the Grammy Foundation). She has authored or co-authored numerous publications, including award-winning journal articles, book chapters, and several books. She is a member of the editorial board of the *Journal of Voice* and is an editorial reviewer for other medical journals, including *Otolaryngology–Head and Neck Surgery*, *The Laryngoscope*, and *Folia Phoniatrica et Logopaedica*.

Robert T. Sataloff, MD, DMA, FACS

Robert T. Sataloff, MD, DMA, FACS is Professor and Chairman, Department of Otolaryngology–Head and Neck Surgery and Senior Associate Dean for Clinical Academic Specialties, Drexel University College of Medicine. He is also Adjunct Professor in the Departments of Otolaryngology–Head and Neck Surgery at Thomas Jefferson University, the University of Pennsylvania, and Temple University; and on the faculty of the Academy of Vocal Arts. Dr. Sataloff is also a professional singer and singing teacher, and he served as Conductor of the Thomas Jefferson University Choir over a period of nearly four decades. He holds an undergraduate degree from Haverford College in Music Theory and Composition; graduated from Jefferson Medical College, Thomas Jefferson University; received a Doctor of Musical Arts in Voice Performance from Combs College of Music; and completed his Residency in Otolaryngology–Head and Neck Surgery and a Fellowship in Otology, Neurotology and Skull Base Surgery at the University of Michigan. Dr. Sataloff is Chairman of the Boards of Directors of the Voice Foundation and of the American Institute for Voice and Ear Research. He has also served as Chairman of the Board of Governors of Graduate Hospital; President of the American Laryngological Association, the International Association of Phonosurgery, and the Pennsylvania Academy of Otolaryngology–Head and Neck Surgery; and in numerous other leadership positions. Dr. Sataloff is Editor-in-Chief of the *Journal of Voice*, Editor-in-Chief of *Ear, Nose and Throat Journal*, Editor-in-Chief of the *Journal of Case Reports in Medicine*, Associate Editor of the *Journal of Singing*, and on the editorial boards of numerous otolaryngology journals. He has written over 1,000 publications, including 42 books. His medical practice is limited to care of the professional voice and to otology/neurotology/skull base surgery.

Mary J. Hawkshaw, BSN, RN, CORLN

Mary J. Hawkshaw, BSN, RN, CORLN is Research Associate Professor in the Department of Otolaryngology–Head and Neck Surgery at Drexel University College of Medicine. She has been associated with Dr. Robert Sataloff, Philadelphia Ear, Nose & Throat Associates, and the American Institute for Voice & Ear Research (AIVER) since 1986. She has served as Secretary/Treasurer of AIVER since 1988 and was named Executive Director of AIVER in January 2000. She has served on the Board of Directors of the Voice Foundation since 1990. Ms. Hawkshaw graduated from Shadyside Hospital School of Nursing in Pittsburgh, PA and received a Bachelor of Science degree in Nursing from Thomas Jefferson University in Philadelphia. In collaboration with Dr. Sataloff, she has co-authored more than 65 book chapters, 160 articles, and 7 textbooks. She is on the Editorial Boards of the *Journal of Voice*; *Ear, Nose and Throat Journal*, and the *Journal of the Society of Otorhinolaryngology and Head-Neck Nurses* (SOHN). She has been an active member of the Society of Otorhinolaryngology and Head-Neck Nurses since 1998. She is recognized nationally and internationally for her extensive contributions to care of the professional voice.

▲ Anatomy: Where is the Voice Produced?

The human voice is remarkable, complex, and delicate. It is capable of conveying not only sophisticated intellectual concepts, but also subtle emotional nuances. Although the uniqueness and beauty of the human voice have been appreciated for centuries, medical scientists have begun to really understand the workings and care of the voice only since the late 1970s and early 1980s. The larynx is the primary organ involved in voice production. However, phonation requires complex interactions between many bodily systems to achieve the sound that we associate with the voice. To fully understand how the voice is produced, it is necessary to understand both the anatomy of the larynx and its neural (nerve) connections, as well as the biomechanics of sound production.

Laryngeal Anatomy

The larynx is the primary source of sound in humans and is commonly referred to as the "voice box." It sits in the neck, just beneath the tongue base and in front of the esophagus, where it serves as the opening to the trachea and lungs (Figure 1-1). In humans, the larynx has four main functions:

- to protect the lungs from foreign materials such as food and liquid,
- to serve as a conduit for the passage of air into the lungs during breathing,
- to produce the voice, and
- to help in stabilizing the pressure within the chest during activities such as lifting and straining.

The larynx is composed of cartilages, muscles, nerves, and the vocal folds. The movements of the vocal folds are coordinated by the actions of the muscles of the larynx, the cartilages of the larynx, and the nerves that supply the muscles of the larynx.[1]

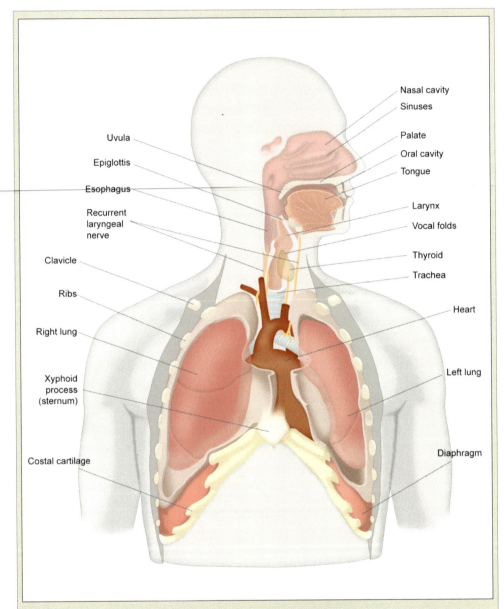

FIGURE 1-1. The respiratory system, showing the relationship between the larynx, the esophagus, the trachea, the lungs, and the diaphragm.

The space between the vocal folds is referred to as the *glottis*, which is the reference point for the vocal tract. Structures within the vocal tract are described as *glottic* (at the level of the vocal folds), *supra*glottic (above the vocal folds), *sub*glottic (just below the vocal folds), or *infra*glottic (well below the vocal folds).

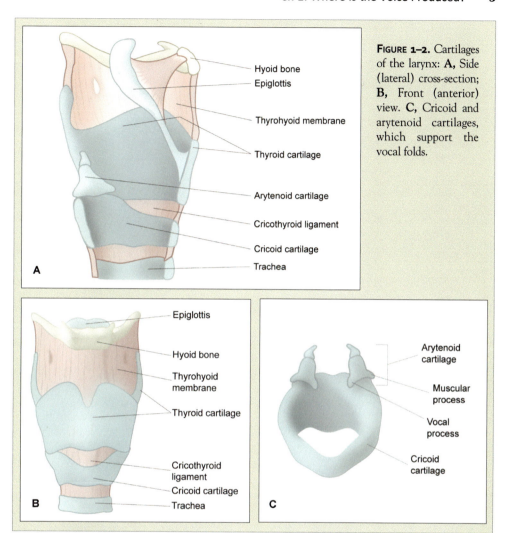

FIGURE 1–2. Cartilages of the larynx: **A,** Side (lateral) cross-section; **B,** Front (anterior) view. **C,** Cricoid and arytenoid cartilages, which support the vocal folds.

LARYNGEAL FRAMEWORK

The laryngeal cartilages provide the structural support for the laryngeal muscles, the vocal folds, and the mucous membranes in a manner similar to the way in which the framework of a house provides support for the walls and floors.

The main cartilages of the larynx are the thyroid, cricoid, arytenoid, and epiglottic cartilages (Figure 1-2A and 2B). At the top of the larynx is the epiglottis, an elastic flap that guards the entrance to the larynx and glottis; it sits upward (open) during breathing and is forced downward (closed) by the tongue during swallowing. The thyroid cartilage below it forms a shield around the upper part of the larynx, providing support and attachment for the laryngeal muscles; it is the familiar "Adam's apple" on the neck.

The cartilages below are important for voice production. The cricoid cartilage forms a ring that provides support for the trachea (Figure 1-2C). The arytenoid car-

4   the Voice

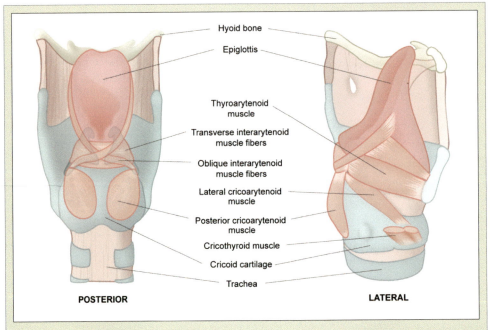

FIGURE 1–3. Intrinsic muscles of the larynx. Back (posterior) and side (lateral) cross-sectional views.

tilages sit on top of the cricoid cartilage. The vocal folds attach to the front edges of the arytenoid cartilages in the back of the larynx and to the thyroid cartilage in the front. The sides and back of the arytenoid cartilages also attach to each of the laryngeal muscles except one, the cricothyroid muscle.

When the laryngeal muscles contract, they move the arytenoid cartilages. Because each arytenoid cartilage is attached to a vocal fold, when the arytenoid cartilages are moved or shifted, the vocal folds are also moved. It is by moving the arytenoid cartilages that the laryngeal muscles are able to move the vocal folds from the opened to closed positions, and vice versa.

The space between the arytenoid cartilage and the cricoid cartilage is the cricoarytenoid joint. This joint has similar characteristics to the knee joint and the joints in the fingers of the hands and feet and is affected similarly by medical conditions that affect other joints in the body. If the cricoarytenoid joint is damaged, the arytenoid cartilage cannot move well, and the mobility of the vocal folds is thus impaired.

LARYNGEAL MUSCLES AND VOCAL FOLDS

The main muscles of the larynx are the thyroarytenoid, posterior cricoarytenoid, lateral cricoarytenoid, interarytenoid, and cricothyroid muscles (Figure 1-3). Each of these muscles is paired, with one located on each side of the larynx. The exception is the interarytenoid muscle, which is a single muscle and sits in the midline of the back of the larynx.

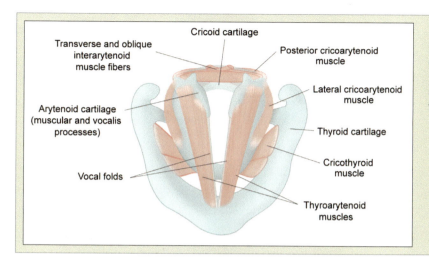

FIGURE 1–4. Muscles and cartilages of the larynx and vocal folds.

The muscles of the larynx function mostly to move the vocal folds by moving the arytenoid, cricoid, and thyroid cartilages (Figure 1-4). They are attached to the cartilages in different locations. It is the location of the attachment of the muscles to the cartilages that determines in which direction the cartilage is pulled.

Together, the thyroarytenoid muscle (part of which is sometimes referred to as the vocalis muscle), its specialized mucosal cover layer (commonly referred to as the mucosal cover or mucosa), and its attachment onto the arytenoid cartilage are referred to as the *vocal fold* (or the true vocal fold). The vocal fold has been referred to also as the "vocal cord," although this term was replaced by the term "vocal fold" in the 1980s because vocal fold is a more accurate description of its shape and structure.

The vocal fold is comprised of five layers of tissue, which create a highly specialized mucosal cover that vibrates to produce the voice (Figure 1-5).[2]

- The deepest layer is the *vocalis muscle* of the vocal fold.
- Overlying the vocalis muscle is thick connective tissue that looks like a ligament or "cord." This tissue has two parts, which scientifically are termed the *deep* and *intermediate layers* of the *lamina propria*. Together, the intermediate and deep layers of the lamina propria comprise the vocal ligament.
- The next layer is the *superficial layer* of lamina propria (sometimes referred to as Reinke's space), which is a gelatinous matrix.
- On top of this matrix lies the *epithelium*, which is the lining tissue and the last (most superficial) layer of the vocal folds, the mucosal cover.

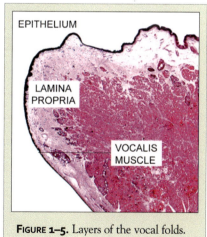

FIGURE 1–5. Layers of the vocal folds.

COURTESY OF J. KOBLER, MASS GENERAL HOSP, BOSTON.

6 *the Voice*

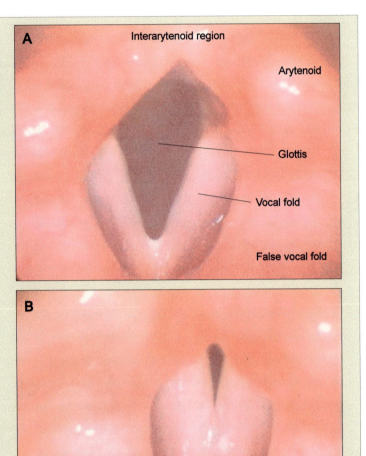

FIGURE 1–6. Vocal folds in open (**A**, normal resting) and closed (**B**, active talking or singing) positions, as seen on rigid strobovideolaryngoscopic examination.

Vibration of the vocal folds during talking and singing occurs when the mucosal cover glides over the gelatinous matrix of the superior lamina propria in a rhythmic fashion.

Normally, during quiet breathing, the vocal folds are open (Figure 1-6A). In order to talk or sing, the muscles in the larynx contract to bring the vocal folds together (Figure 1-6B). Air from the lungs causes the mucosal cover of the vocal folds to glide sideways over the vocal ligament, resulting in a slight escape of air past the "closed" vocal folds. The mucosal cover then glides back to completely close the space between the vocal folds, and this cycle (which is sometimes referred to as the *vibratory cycle*) repeats itself (Figure 1-7). This gliding of the mucosal cover back and forth is the vibration of the vocal folds that produces the voice.

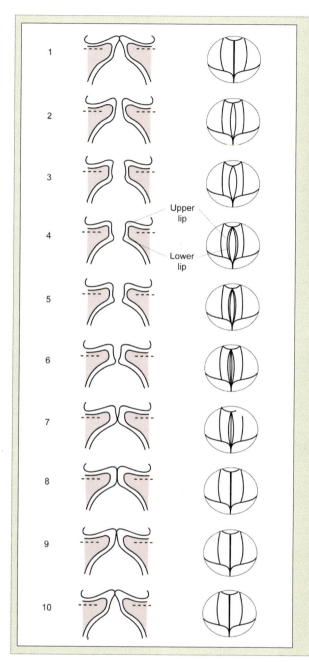

FIGURE 1–7. Vibration of the vocal folds, during the production of a sound, is shown in a cross-section through the middle part of the vocal folds (*left column*) and from above the vocal folds (*right column*). Just before separation, the vocal folds are completely closed (*1*). The mucosal cover glides open and then closes (*2-6*), revealing a slight phase difference between the upper and lower lips (surfaces) of the vocal fold. The inferior lip closes first (*7*) and opens first (*9-10*) as air flows from the lungs to repeat the vibratory cycle.

When the cricothyroid muscle contracts, it tenses the vocal fold (Figure 1-8A).[1] Tensing the vocal fold stretches it, making it longer and thinner. Like the strings on a piano, longer, thinner vocal folds produce a high pitch, and shorter, thicker vocal folds produce a low pitch. Whereas the cricothyroid muscles contract to stretch and thin the vocal folds to raise the pitch of the voice, it is the thyroarytenoid muscle (Figure 1-8B) that contracts to shorten and thicken the vocal

FIGURE 1–8. Actions of the intrinsic muscles of the larynx. **A,** When the cricothyroid muscles contract (*red arrow*), they pull the front part of the cricoid cartilage upwards (*blue arrow*), toward the thyroid cartilage, causing the vocal ligaments to stretch and raising the pitch of the voice. **B,** In the bottom four panels, the directional arrows suggest muscle actions and their resulting effects on the vocal ligaments and glottis opening.

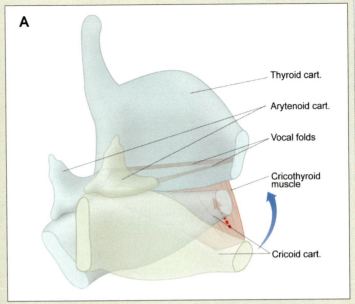

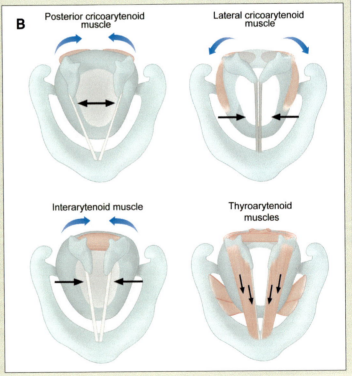

folds to create a lower pitch. When the posterior cricoarytenoid muscle contracts, it pulls the vocal folds open and allows air to enter the lungs during breathing. This action also occurs intermittently during phonation to allow breaks between sounds.

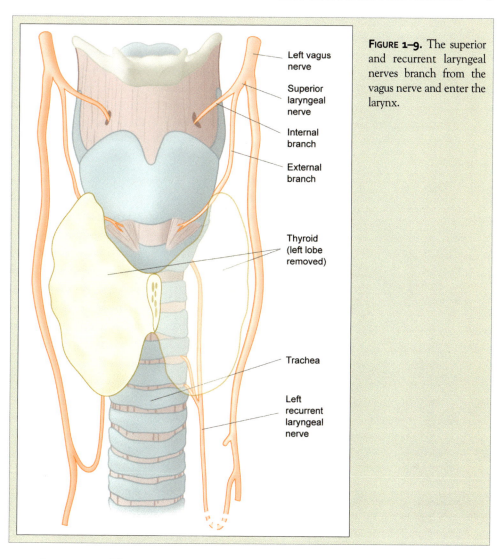

FIGURE 1–9. The superior and recurrent laryngeal nerves branch from the vagus nerve and enter the larynx.

LARYNGEAL NERVES

The larynx has two sets of nerves, the superior laryngeal nerves and the recurrent laryngeal nerves (Figure 1-9). In general, nerves can either send messages to muscles from the brain to initiate movement or they can take messages to the brain from the body with information regarding sensation, pain, and temperature. Nerves that initiate movement are termed motor nerves. Those that carry information regarding sensation are termed sensory nerves.

The superior laryngeal nerve supplies motor function to the cricothyroid muscle and carries sensory information from the vocal folds and the parts of the larynx above the vocal folds. The recurrent laryngeal nerve supplies motor function to the remaining muscles of the larynx and carries sensory information from the vocal folds and the parts of the larynx below the vocal folds.

Details of the anatomy are summarized below. They may seem a bit complicated for the average voice professional, but the information is invaluable for anyone contemplating surgery in or around the larynx, neck, or chest (such as thyroidectomy, for example) or for anyone who wants to understand the vocal instrument well enough to master the craft of using the voice or teaching others to use it.

The recurrent laryngeal nerve and superior laryngeal nerve are branches of the vagus nerve (the tenth cranial nerve). Each of these sets of nerves is paired, with one of the pair on each side of the neck and larynx. The vagus nerve begins in the brainstem, the portion of the brain at the base of the skull. The vagus nerve exits the base of the skull and enters the neck, where its laryngeal component branches twice (Figure 1-9).

The superior laryngeal nerve is the first branch. The superior laryngeal nerve has two branches, an internal and an external branch. The internal branch enters the larynx through the thyrohyoid membrane, just above the thyroid cartilage. The internal branch carries sensory information from the vocal folds and the portions of the larynx above the vocal folds to the brain, where that information is integrated to produce a perception of sensation.

The external branch of the superior laryngeal nerve supplies motor function to the cricothyroid muscle. The external branch descends in the neck with the superior thyroid artery, courses over the upper pole of the thyroid gland, and enters the cricothyroid muscle, where it helps to control pitch and inflection in the voice. Because of its association with the upper pole of the thyroid gland, this nerve can be easily injured during thyroid surgery from stretching and manipulation of the gland.

After the superior laryngeal nerve branches, the vagus nerve travels into the chest to supply neural innervation to the heart, where it helps regulate heart rate and blood pressure. In the chest, the recurrent laryngeal nerve separates from the vagus nerve, swings under the arch of the aorta on the left and under the brachial artery on the right, and returns back into the neck (hence, the name "recurrent") (Figure 1-9). In the neck, the nerve travels in the groove formed by the abutment of the trachea on the esophagus and on the undersurface of the thyroid gland.

Underneath the thyroid gland, the recurrent laryngeal nerve enters the larynx behind the cricothyroid joint and supplies motor function to the thyroarytenoid, interarytenoid, posterior cricoarytenoid, and lateral cricoarytenoid muscles. The recurrent laryngeal nerve also carries sensory information as discussed above.

There is some rejoining of fibers of the recurrent laryngeal nerve and the internal branch of the superior laryngeal nerves within the thyroarytenoid muscle, implying that there may be some cross-over function between the two branches and that the potential exists for one of the nerves to compensate when damage occurs to the other.

Because of the long route of the recurrent laryngeal nerves from the brain, through the neck, into the chest, and back to the larynx, there exists a large potential for injury from blunt or penetrating trauma to the chest or neck and from a variety of surgical procedures. The nerves are most commonly injured during surgical procedures to the thyroid, parathyroid, heart, lung, chest, carotid, cervical spine, and vertebral arteries, but can be injured by any surgery that is performed near the nerve in the head, neck, or chest.[3]

When the nerve is partially injured from stretching, swelling, or manipulation during surgery, paresis (partial weakness) of the vocal fold results. This is discussed in detail in Chapter 10. If the nerve is cut, vocal fold paralysis (complete weakness, rather than partial) usually results.

How Do the Brain and Nerves Interact to Produce the Voice?

Voice production is extremely complex. Voluntary production of the voice begins in the brain. Production of the voice begins with a thought that essentially tells the brain "I want to produce a sound." This thought is then conveyed into a command that tells the body to do all the things necessary to produce the voice.

The command and the thought are produced in two separate regions of the brain. The command involves a complex matrix of interactions among the brain centers for speech and other areas in the cerebral cortex. For singing, the commands for speech must be integrated with information from the centers in the brain that control musical and artistic expression.

The thought is conveyed to an area of the brain termed the precentral gyrus. The precentral gyrus is located in the motor cortex, which is the portion of the brain that controls all muscle functions in the body. The precentral gyrus transmits another set of instructions to the brainstem and spinal cord. These areas send out the complicated messages necessary for coordinated activity of the muscles in the larynx, chest, abdomen, back, and vocal tract.

These impulses combine to produce a sound that is transmitted not only to the ears of the listener, but also to those of the speaker or singer. Feedback from the ears of the speaker/singer is transmitted back through the brainstem to the cerebral cortex, and adjustments are made that permit the vocalist to match the sound produced with the sound intended. Sensory feedback, such as the feeling that one is projecting into the head or chest, also helps in the fine tuning of vocal output, although the mechanism and role of sensory feedback is not fully understood. Many trained singers and speakers learn to use sensory feedback effectively because of expected interference with auditory feedback data from ancillary sound, such as an orchestra, choir, or band.

How do the Framework, Muscles, and Nerves Interact to Produce the Voice?

The vocal folds act as the oscillator or sound source (noise maker) of the vocal tract. The intrinsic muscles of the larynx alter the position, shape, and tension of the vocal folds, bringing them together, moving them apart, or stretching them by increasing longitudinal tension. They are able to do so because the laryngeal cartilages are connected by soft attachments that allow changes in their relative angles and distances, thereby permitting alteration in the shape and tension of the tissues suspended between them. The arytenoid cartilages are also capable of rocking, rotating, and gliding, which permits complex vocal fold motion and alteration in the shape of the vocal fold edge.

Because the attachments of the laryngeal cartilages are flexible, the positions of the cartilages change with respect to each other when the laryngeal skeleton is elevated or lowered. Such changes in vertical height are controlled by the extrinsic laryngeal muscles, or strap muscles of the neck.

When the angles and distances between cartilages change because of this accordion effect, the resulting length of the intrinsic muscles is also changed. Such large adjustments in intrinsic muscle condition interfere with fine control of smooth vocal quality. This is why classically trained singers are generally taught to use their extrinsic muscles to maintain the laryngeal skeleton at a relatively constant height regardless of pitch. That is, they learn to avoid the natural tendency of the larynx to rise with ascending pitch and fall with descending pitch, thereby enhancing unity of quality throughout the vocal range. Techniques may be different in certain Asian, Indian, Arabic, and other musical traditions with different aesthetic values.

VOCAL FOLD LUBRICATION

The vocal folds need adequate lubrication to maintain healthy vibration, particularly with prolonged phonation. This is achieved best by ensuring that the body is well hydrated at all times, but particularly prior to performing.

Hydration is accomplished by drinking water or drinks that have balanced electrolytes, such as Gatorade™. Urine color is a good guide to the state of hydration. A pale urine color implies that there is adequate hydration for the kidneys, which usually is a good sign of adequate hydration throughout the body. Those with known kidney disorders, heart disease, hypertension, pituitary abnormalities, adrenal gland dysfunction, and other health problems should consult their physician and exercise caution before attempting to maintain hydration in this manner, as these individuals' usual mechanisms for fluid control may be impaired.

Water is preferred over juices or concentrated beverages. The sugar, salts, and sweeteners in such drinks limit the amount of water that is absorbed by the body. Caffeinated beverages and alcohol are dehydrating and should be avoided during and for several days prior to vocal performance. It is most ideal for the busy voice to be hydrated at all times to prevent rapid changes in the body's fluid content. Because of the concern for reflux during performances, large quantities of liquid/water should not be consumed within the 2 hours prior to or during vocal performance.

Summary

The primary source for voice production in the human body is the larynx. The larynx houses the vocal folds, which vibrate to produce the voice when air is blown past them from the lungs. Coordination between muscles in the larynx, signals from the brain, and muscles in the abdomen, back, chest, head, and neck help with fine tuning of the signal to produce the sound that we associate with the voice.

References

1. Sataloff RT. The human voice. *Scientific American* 1992; 267(6):108–115.
2. Hirano M. Structure and vibratory pattern of the vocal folds. In: Sawashima N, Cooper FS, eds. *Dynamic Aspects of Speech Production*. Tokyo: University of Tokyo Press; 1977: pp13–27.
3. Heman-Ackah YD, Batory M. Determining the cause of mild vocal fold hypomobility. *Journal of Voice* 2003; 17(4):579–588.

▲ How is the Voice Produced?

The Mechanics of Voice Production

Production of the voice involves the same physics as the mechanism of sound production from any source, such as a musical instrument. In general, the production of sound requires four main components:

- airflow
- an oscillator (an instrument that puts the airflow into a wave-like motion, thus creating sound waves)
- a resonator (which helps to maintain a uniform frequency of vibration), and
- an amplifier (which increases the magnitude of the sound waves to make them louder).

In the case of the trumpet, power is generated by the chest, abdomen, and back musculature, and a high-pressure air stream is produced. The trumpeter's lips open and close against the mouthpiece, producing a "buzz" similar to the sound produced by vocal fold vibration. This sound then passes through the trumpet, whose twisted shape creates a resonance chamber that shapes the sound and gives it its "signature." This "signature" helps us identify the sound as coming from a trumpet and not a flute or clarinet, for example. The resonance chamber of the trumpet is analogous to the vocal tract, which acts as a biological resonance chamber.

In voice production, the source of airflow is the lungs. The abdominal, diaphragm, chest, and back musculatures contribute to airflow in voice production. The oscillator is the vocal folds, which vibrate and place the airflow into a wave-like motion. The remainder of the vocal tract, the supraglottic larynx, the pharynx (throat), the oral cavity (mouth) including the lips, tongue and palate, the nasal cavity, the sinuses, and the head together form the resonance chamber and amplifier for voice production in humans (Figure 2-1).

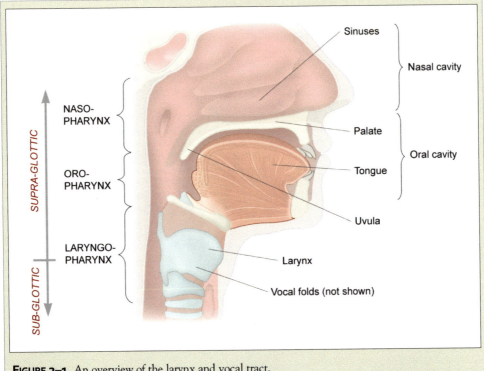

FIGURE 2–1. An overview of the larynx and vocal tract.

Sound Source

The sound source for voice production is the larynx and the vibrating vocal folds. The vocal folds themselves are made of five layers of tissue, as explained in Chapter 1.

The outer mucosa (epithelium) forms the thin, lubricated surface of the vocal folds, which makes contact when the two vocal folds are closed. It looks like the mucosa lining the inside of the mouth. Mechanically, however, the vocal fold structures act more like three layers, consisting of the mucosal cover layer (epithelium and superficial layer of the lamina propria), the transition layer (intermediate and deep layers of the lamina propria), and the body (the vocalis muscle).

When one makes the decision to talk, the vocal folds come together in the midline (Figure 2-2A). Air is forced from the lungs past the closed vocal folds. The epithelium of the vocal folds glides open, over the superficial layer of lamina propria. As the mucosal cover opens, air travels past the vocal folds and into the upper parts of the larynx and pharynx. A Bernoulli force, similar to a "suction effect," is created by the air that passes between the vocal folds (Figure 2-2B). This Bernoulli force combines with the mechanical properties of the vocal folds to begin closing the lower portion of the vocal folds almost immediately, even while the upper edges are still separating.

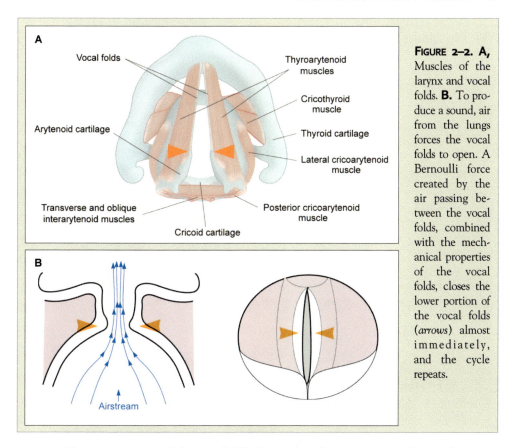

FIGURE 2–2. **A,** Muscles of the larynx and vocal folds. **B.** To produce a sound, air from the lungs forces the vocal folds to open. A Bernoulli force created by the air passing between the vocal folds, combined with the mechanical properties of the vocal folds, closes the lower portion of the vocal folds (*arrows*) almost immediately, and the cycle repeats.

The upper portion of the vocal folds has strong elastic properties that tend to make the vocal folds snap back to the midline. The upper portions of the vocal folds are then returned to the closed position, completing the glottic cycle. When the vocal folds snap shut, sound (i.e., a sound wave) is produced.[1] Subglottal pressure then builds again, and the events repeat.

The frequency of opening and closing of the vocal folds (the vibratory cycle) determines the frequency of the sound waves and, thus, the pitch of the voice. The frequency of the vibratory cycle is dependent on the strength of the airflow from the lungs and on mechanical properties of the vocal folds, which are regulated in part by the laryngeal muscles. Under most circumstances, as the vocal folds are thinned and stretched and airflow is increased, the frequency of air pulse emission increases, and pitch goes up.

The frequency of vibration of the vocal folds is termed the *fundamental frequency*, and the character of the sound that is produced from the vocal folds is very similar to the sound that is produced from buzzing lips.[2] This is a complex sound containing a fundamental frequency and many overtones, or higher harmonic partials. The amplitude (which determines volume) of the harmonic partials decreases uniformly at approximately 12 decibels (dB) per octave. This complex sound is modified by the resonance chamber of the supraglottic vocal tract and produces the voice that gives each person his or her own characteristic and distinguishing vocal signature.[3]

A louder sound can be produced by one of three methods: 1) by increasing the airflow from the lungs, 2) by increasing glottal resistance, or 3) by changing the shape of the vocal tract. The preferred method of increasing volume is to increase airflow from the lungs, along with changing the shape of the palate, mouth, and oral cavity to facilitate amplification and projection of the voice. Greater forces of air streaming from the lungs cause the epithelium of the vocal folds to be pushed farther apart and more air rushes between them. The vocal folds are able to snap together more abruptly, creating a louder sound. When less airflow is used from the lungs, the vocal folds are blown apart to a lesser degree and a softer sound is produced.

Clapping the hands can mimic this effect somewhat. When the hands are wide apart at the start of each clap, a louder sound is produced. When the hands are closer together at the start of each clap, a softer sound is produced.

The vocal folds function in a similar fashion. In order to raise the volume by increasing the glottal resistance, the individual forcefully closes the vocal folds. Oftentimes, doing so involves recruiting the accessory muscles of phonation, including the pharyngeal constrictors, the strap muscles in the neck, and the base of the tongue, as well as using the vocal folds themselves. Such use of excess force is termed *laryngeal hyperfunction*, and the forceful closure of the vocal folds can cause vocal fold trauma resulting in vocal fold tears, hemorrhages, edema (swelling), or masses such as nodules, polyps, or cysts.

If the vocal folds cannot close completely, a space exists between them during speaking and singing. This gap can be caused by a mild vocal fold paresis, vocal fold masses (such as a polyp, nodule, or cyst), vocal fold scar, or vocal fold swelling, resulting in an escape of air throughout the phonatory cycle and inability of the epithelium of the vocal folds to close completely consistently (Figure 2-3). Thus, the same degree of effort from the lungs produces a softer, breathier sounding voice.

A somewhat similar effect can be demonstrated by cupping the hands in a C-shaped fashion so that when the hands are clapped together, there is always a space between the palms. If the hands open with the same degree of excursion as they did uncupped, a softer clap is produced. To produce the same loudness of clapping with the hands cupped as with them uncupped, the cupped hands need to have a wider degree of excursion and more forceful closure with each clap than do the uncupped hands.

From a voice perspective, when a gap exists between the vocal folds, this translates into a greater requirement for increased airflow from the lungs than is needed when the vocal folds are perfectly symmetric and meet in the midline. From a functional perspective, incomplete vocal fold closure often translates into a softer, breathy voice, increased phonatory effort, greater vocal fatigue, and increased vocal strain with prolonged voice use. More energy is needed to produce greater airflow from the lungs to increase volume and projection and to sustain phonation, which creates a greater susceptibility to fatigue. Because of this greater susceptibility to fatigue, many people with incomplete glottic closure subconsciously compensate by recruiting the accessory muscles of phonation, and then begin to suffer the consequences of laryngeal hyperfunction as well as those associated with incomplete closure.

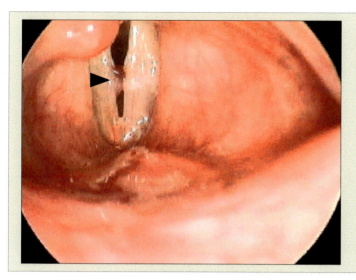

FIGURE 2–3. A vocal fold mass (*arrow*) inhibiting complete closure of the vocal folds.

Resonance and Amplification

The resonance chamber and amplifier of the voice is the supraglottic vocal tract, which includes the back of the nose and throat (nasopharynx), the tongue, the palate, the mouth, the sinuses, and the head (*see* Figure 2-1).

The pharynx, oral cavity, and nasal cavity act as a series of interconnected resonators, which are more complex than that in the trumpet example or other single resonators. The vocal tract resonators determine (in part) vocal quality. A resonator is any system that has weight and that can be compressed.[3]

As with other resonators, some frequencies are attenuated (dampened), while others are enhanced. Enhanced frequencies are then radiated with higher relative amplitudes (intensities). This attenuation and enhancement occurs as a result of sound waves bouncing back and forth against the walls of the vocal tract. As the sound resonates throughout the vocal tract, it gains energy at those frequencies that are amplified by the particular shape of the vocal tract and loses energy in those areas that are dampened by the shape of the vocal tract.[3] Because everyone's pharynx, oral cavity, nasopharynx, and head are shaped differently, amplification of the fundamental frequencies occurs in different patterns from one person to another.

The frequencies with high energy are termed the *harmonic frequencies* and occur at multiples of the fundamental frequency.[3] Some harmonic frequencies are amplified and others are dampened by the resonating properties of the vocal tract. The harmonic frequencies are responsible for giving each voice its own "signature" sound that allows us to distinguish one individual from another. The harmonic frequencies also give the voice its "ring," which allows the voice to be heard even in the presence of significant background noise.[3] Changing the shape of the vocal tract by altering the position of the tongue, the shape of the pharynx, and the position of the palate changes the characteristics of the harmonics and, thus, the projection and volume achieved.[3]

The vocal tract has four or five important harmonic frequencies called *formants*.[3] The singer's formant is of special interest. It has a strong acoustical peak at about 2,400 to 3,200 Hz, depending on voice classification. It is responsible for the "ring" that allows a solo singer to be heard over the sounds of choirs, orchestras, and environmental noise. Even though it is roughly 3 ½ octaves above middle C, it is an essential component of a singer's sound. If it is filtered out, even a great voice like that of Pavarotti will lose its ring and disappear into the surrounding envelope of sound. While a stronger singer's formant is essential for easy, exciting solo singing, it is not always a blessing in choral singers. This energy peak must be adjusted and managed to prevent strong voices from standing out in a choral setting.

Amplification of the voice occurs primarily in the oral cavity, which has a megaphone-like effect on vocal projection. A more open mouth and oral cavity causes greater intensity of the voice as it leaves the body. This is achieved best by focusing on the position of the tongue and its base, the palate, and the lips. Elongation and widening of the vocal tract are accomplished using several conscious mechanisms, including maintaining correct neck posture. If the neck is tilted back or the chin is lifted too high, a bend is created in the pharyngeal area, which effectively narrows the resonance chamber at the region of the tongue base. The head usually should be in a neutral position so that the spine is straight through the skull base.[3] This produces a straighter vocal tract and enhances resonance and projection.

Elevation of the palate helps to open the resonance tract in the back of the oral cavity and seals the nasopharynx to minimize hypernasality. Relaxation of the tongue base, with the tip of the tongue resting in a more forward position, helps to lengthen the oral cavity and widen the space at the tongue base, creating a longer, greater diameter amplifier.[3]

Airflow and Breathing

The infraglottic vocal tract (below the larynx) serves as the power source for the voice. Singers and actors refer to the entire power source complex as their "support" or "diaphragm." Actually, the anatomy of support for phonation is especially complicated and not completely understood. Performers who use the terms *diaphragm* and *support* do not always mean the same thing. Yet, it is quite important because deficiencies in support are frequently responsible for voice dysfunction.

The purpose of the support mechanism is to generate a force that directs a controlled air stream between the vocal folds. Airflow for vocal production involves a complex interplay between the lungs, the abdomen, the chest, the back, the legs and hips, as well as the brain, ears, and balance organs. Active respiratory muscles work together with passive forces. The principal muscles of inspiration (inhalation) are the diaphragm (a dome-shaped muscle that extends along the bottom of the rib cage) and the external intercostal (rib) muscles. During quiet breathing,

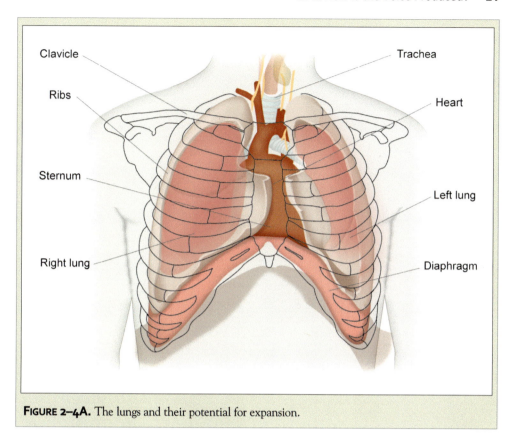

FIGURE 2–4A. The lungs and their potential for expansion.

expiration (exhalation) is largely passive, meaning that it occurs without significant muscular effort. The lungs and rib cage generate passive expiratory forces under many common circumstances, such as after a full breath.

The Lungs

The lungs have the ability to expand in all three dimensions, with the greatest potential for excursion being down (Figure 2-4A). The lungs are housed within the chest cavity, are separated from the abdomen by the diaphragm, and are encased on all sides by the ribs. The ribs limit the amount of outward expansion of the lungs, leaving the greatest room for expansion down into the abdomen.[4] The diaphragm contracts (moves down) with inhalation and relaxes (moves up) with exhalation.[5] As the diaphragm contracts with inhalation, the abdominal contents are pushed downward and outward to allow room for the expanding lungs.

During normal, resting-state respiration, exhalation is largely passive.[5] The diaphragm relaxes as air is released from the lungs. With active exhalation, the abdominal muscles contract and the diaphragm relaxes as air is forced out of the lungs.[5] This increases the negative pressure in the chest, creating a suction effect.

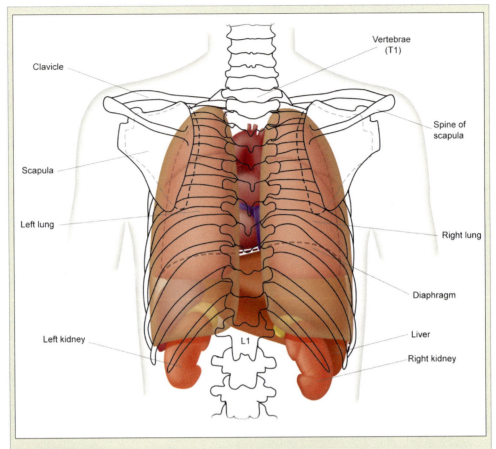

FIGURE 2–4B. Back view of the lungs, showing their potential for expansion.

As the abdominal muscles relax and the diaphragm contracts into the abdomen, more air is siphoned into the lungs with the inhalation. Larger and controlled breaths employ both the diaphragm and abdomen for breathing, and shallow breaths use diaphragmatic breathing only. In voice production, greater control of airflow, and thus the voice, can be achieved with breathing strategies that incorporate efficient use of abdominal and back muscles.

The right lung is divided into three lobes, while the left lung is divided into two lobes only. Each lobe functions much like a balloon, expanding when air enters during inhalation and shrinking when air leaves during exhalation.[5] Like balloons, the lobes of the lung have a certain degree of elasticity, which allows this expansion and recoil. The lower lobes of the lungs have the capacity for the greatest volume, and also have the greatest compliance, which allows for greater expansion into the abdomen.[5]

The ribs surround the upper lobes of the lungs, thus limiting their ability to expand and recoil. The positioning of the collarbones and the scapulae (shoulder blades) also limits the expansion of the lungs. The optimal position for expansion is with both the collarbones and scapulae flat, down, and maximally expanded horizontally, to allow for maximal pulmonary expansion and filling (Figure 2-4B).

Many of the muscles used for active expiration are also employed in "support" for phonation. Muscles of active expiration either raise the intraabdominal pressure forcing the diaphragm upward, or lower the ribs and sternum (breast bone) to decrease the dimensions of the thorax, or both, thereby compressing air in the chest. The primary muscles of expiration are the "abdominal muscles," but internal intercostal (rib) and other chest and back muscles also are involved. Trauma or surgery that alters the structure or function of these muscles or ribs undermines the power source of the voice, as do diseases that impair expiration, such as asthma.

Deficiencies in the support mechanism often result in compensatory efforts that strain the laryngeal muscles, which are not designed for power source functions. Such behavior can result in decreased voice function, rapid fatigue, pain, and even structural pathology including vocal fold nodules. Currently, expert treatment (voice therapy) for such problems focuses on correction of the underlying malfunction. This often cures the problem, avoiding the need for laryngeal surgery.

The compliance of the lungs can be limited further by obstructive lung diseases, such as asthma and chronic obstructive pulmonary disease (from smoking). In such cases, the lungs are able to inhale the same amount of air; however, the force produced on exhalation is drastically reduced due to the limited recoil within the lungs. Restrictive lung diseases, such as emphysema and the effects of broken ribs, limit the amount of air the lungs can inhale and thus the amount of air the lungs can exhale. Each of these then affects airflow and control during voice production and can predispose to vocal hyperfunction, fatigue, decreased vocal projection, and vocal injury.

The Abdomen

The abdomen contributes to breathing by helping to produce a suction effect on the diaphragm and lungs. The abdomen consists of several layers of muscles: the external oblique, the internal oblique, the transverse abdominus, and the rectus abdominus muscles (Figure 2-5).

The *external oblique* muscles lie immediately beneath the skin and fat. They insert into and obtain their strength during contraction from a central, dense layer of tissue (the fascial insertion). The *internal oblique* muscles lie beneath the external oblique muscles and run horizontally along the side of the abdomen. Much of the abdominal contribution to breathing is from the internal and external obliques.[6]

The *rectus abdominus* muscles lie in the center of the abdomen with their fibers running vertically. The rectus abdominus muscle bends the torso when it contracts. Its main function is to support the back and to assist with balance; it does not contribute much to breathing.

Under the internal oblique muscles lie the *transverse abdominal* muscles (not visible in Figure 2-5), which contribute little to breathing and breath support and more

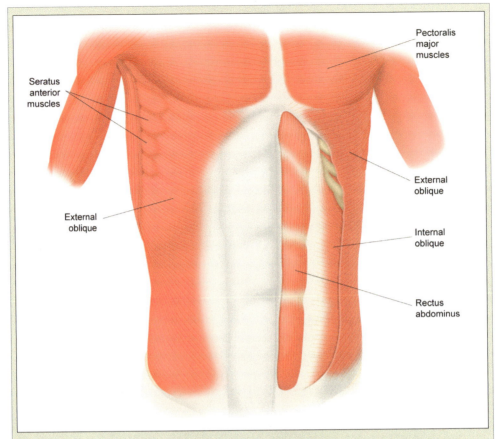

FIGURE 2–5. The abdominal muscles, showing the superficial layers on the left and the deep layers on the right.

to core strengthening. Sustained contraction of the abdomen during exhalation helps to regulate the flow of air from the lungs during breathing and phonation.

Knowledge of abdominal anatomy and musculature is critical for the voice professional who is considering abdominal surgery and very helpful to anyone trying to understand breathing or "support." Surgery on the abdomen weakens the muscles that are cut. Rehabilitation and strengthening of the weakened abdominal muscles prior to resuming a normal vocal routine is imperative for the professional voice user in helping to prevent vocal injury, even in the most trained voice professional.

The Back

The back consists of five to six layers of muscles whose fibers cross each other (Figure 2-6). The main function of the back is to help maintain balance and to

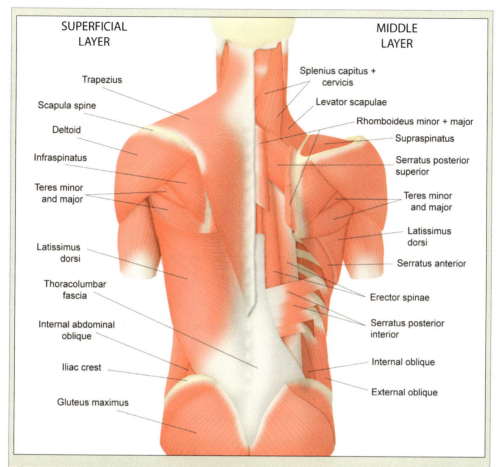

FIGURE 2–6. The back muscles, showing the superficial layers on the left and the middle layers on the right.

serve as a support for the abdomen. Abdominal support of breathing requires the support of the back muscles to maximize the force of any given abdominal contractile effort. If firm support from the back occurs simultaneously with pressure from the abdomen, a greater force is created.

Summary

Voice production results from the interplay between airflow, oscillation, resonance, and amplification. Many organ systems in the body participate actively in phonation in addition to the larynx, and each has a vital role. The vocal mechanism includes the larynx, the abdominal and back musculature, the rib cage, the lungs, and the pharynx, oral cavity, and nose. Each component performs an important function in voice production.

Knowledge of the physiology of voice production, as well as of the anatomy of the organs that contribute to voice production, is the first step in understanding how to care for and maintain the voice throughout one's professional career.

References

1. Sataloff RT. Clinical anatomy and physiology of the voice. In: Sataloff RT. *Professional Voice: The Science and Art of Clinical Care*, 3rd ed. San Diego: Plural Publications; 2005: pp143–178.
2. Sundberg J. The acoustics of the singing voice. *Scientific American* 1977; 236 (6):82–91.
3. Sundberg J. Vocal tract resonance. In: Sataloff RT. *Professional Voice: The Science and Art of Clinical Care*, 3rd ed. San Diego: Plural Publications; 2005: pp275–292.
4. Gould WJ, Okamura H. Static lung volumes in singers. *Annals of Otology Rhinology and Laryngology* 1973; 82:89–95.
5. West JB. Mechanics of breathing. In: West JB, ed. *Best and Taylor's Physiological Basis of Medical Practice*, 11th ed. Baltimore: Williams & Wilkins; 1985: pp586–604.
6. Hixon TJ, Hoffman C. Chest wall shape during singing. In: Lawrence V, ed. *Transcripts of the Seventh Annual Symposium, Care of the Professional Voice*. New York: The Voice Foundation; 1978: pp9–10.

▲ How Do I Maintain Longevity of My Voice?

3

Those who use their voice professionally for singing, acting, teaching, counseling, public speaking, telecommunications, oration, or other venues need to maintain good vocal hygiene to sustain reliable, lifelong professional voice use. Like dental hygiene, vocal hygiene is a set of preventative measures that are actively and consciously undertaken by the voice user to maintain the health, reliability, and consistency of the voice. Proper training, strengthening, and conditioning are as important to the professional voice user as they are to a professional athlete.[1] Attention to these practices will help prevent vocal injury and maintain the voice through rigorous vocal performance and speaking schedules.

How Can The Voice Be Kept Healthy?

Preventative medicine is always the best medicine. The more one understands his or her voice, the more one will appreciate its importance and delicacy. Education helps us understand how to protect the voice, train and develop it to handle our individual vocal demands, and keep it healthy. A little bit of expert voice training can make a big difference.

Avoidance of abuses, especially smoke, is paramount. If voice problems occur, expert medical care with a laryngologist (an ear, nose, and throat doctor who specializes in voice care) should be sought promptly. Interdisciplinary collaboration among laryngologists, speech-language pathologists, singing teachers, acting teachers, many other professionals, and especially voice users themselves has revolutionized voice care since the early 1980s.[1] Technological advances, scientific revelations, and new medical techniques inspired by interest in professional opera singers have brought a new level of expertise and concern to the medical profession and improved dramatically the level of care available for any patient with voice dysfunction.

How Can A "Normal" Voice Be Made Better?

Voice building is possible, productive, and extremely gratifying. Speaking and singing are athletic. They involve muscle strength, endurance, and coordination. Like any other athletic endeavor, voice use is enhanced by training that includes exercises designed to build strength and coordination throughout the vocal tract. Speaking is so natural that the importance of training is not always obvious. However, running is just as natural. Yet, most people recognize that, no matter how well a person runs, he or she will run better and faster under the tutelage of a good track coach. The coach will also provide instruction on strengthening and warm-up and cool-down exercises that prevent injury. Voice training works similarly.

Voice building starts with physical development. Once vocal health has been assured by medical examination, training is usually guided by a voice trainer (with schooling in theater and acting voice techniques), singing teacher, or a speech-language pathologist. In the authors' setting, all three specialists are involved under the guidance of a laryngologist (the voice doctor), and additional voice team members are utilized, as well, including a psychologist or psychiatrist (for stress-management), pulmonologist, neurologist, and others.

Initially, training focuses on the development of physical strength, endurance, and coordination. This is accomplished not only through vocal exercises but also through medically supervised bodily exercise that improve aerobic conditioning and strength in the support system. Singing skills are developed (even in people with virtually no singing talent at all) and used to enhance speech quality, variability, projection, and stamina. For most people, marked voice improvement occurs quickly. For those with particularly challenging vocal needs, voice building also includes training and coordinating body language with vocal messages, organizing presentations, managing adversarial situations (interviews, court appearances, etc.), television performance techniques, and other skills that make the difference between a good professional voice user and a great one.

The process of voice building is valuable not just for premier professional voice users. Virtually all of us depend upon our voices to convey our personalities and ideas. The right subliminal vocal messages can be as important in selling a product or getting a job as they are in convincing a jury or winning a presidential election. The initial stages of voice building are no more complex than the initial stages of learning to play tennis or golf, and their potential value is unlimited. A strong, confident, well-modulated voice quietly commands attention, convinces, and conveys a message of health, strength, youth and credibility.

Care of the Conversational Voice

The source of many voice problems in both professional speakers and professional singers lies in unrecognized abuse or misuse of the everyday speaking voice. Such misuse and abuse can take the form of chronic throat clearing, yelling or shouting above loud noises, or engaging in prolonged or emotionally charged conversations without paying attention to breath support, resonance, or proper body alignment. Even for the best trained voice professional, it is easy to forget to employ proper vocal techniques during normal conversation, and conscious efforts must be made to use these techniques at all times. Otherwise, the larynx may be subjected to phonotrauma, which may lead to the development of nodules, polyps, cysts, or hemorrhage (bleeding) on the vocal folds and a resultant hoarse voice.[2]

The voice should always be *warmed-up* at the start of each day, prior to talking, and *cooled-down* at bedtime. Vocal warm-ups and cool-downs are analogous to stretching exercises used with other muscle groups. In the morning, they help to prepare the vocal muscles for prolonged use: that is, a day of conversational speech.

- The warm-up exercises used should include exercises in pitch variation to help stretch and tone the tensor muscles of the vocal folds, as well as exercises to help stretch and tone the opening and closing muscles of the larynx.[3] In addition, exercises that focus on proper breathing and control of respiration during phonation should be employed to help tone the abdominal muscles and prepare them for use in support of phonation.[3] Exercises to help relax the accessory muscles of phonation, such as stretching and loosening the tongue, lips, jaw, shoulder, and neck, should be performed at the beginning of the warm-up. Exercises designed to recruit the appropriate muscles in the vocal tract for the production of an optimal resonance pattern should be employed each morning. The focus of such exercises should be forward placement of the voice.
- The cool-down exercises should also stretch the muscles that tense, close, and open the vocal folds, but the focus here is not to increase tone but rather to help the vocal muscles achieve a state of healthy relaxation after a day of prolonged use.

All of the exercises chosen should be taught by and practiced initially with a voice teacher or speech-language pathologist who specializes in voice care (often referred to as a voice pathologist or voice therapist). These individuals help to provide objective feedback and ensure that the exercises are being done safely and correctly. Just as improper technique while weight-lifting without a trainer can result in a muscle tear or strain, so can the improper performance of vocal exercises without proper guidance.

The prevention of harmful muscle use patterns during conversational speech helps to limit the development of vocal fold masses, such as polyps, nodules, and cysts. Voice misuse (incorrect voice technique) and voice abuse (harmful behaviors that damage the vocal folds, such as yelling or screaming) can cause both acute and chronic vocal fold injury. Yelling and screaming, particularly during emotionally charged situations, and talking over loud noise can cause forceful closure of the vocal folds, which can result in vocal fold hemorrhage (bleeding) (Figure 3-1), the development of "blisters" in the form of polyps (Figure 3-2) or cysts (Figure 3-3), or the formation of nodules (Figure 3-4), the laryngeal equivalent of callouses.

For those who need to project their voice over loud noises (for example, stock brokers, politicians, machinists, construction workers, or cheerleaders, to name a few), working with a voice teacher or voice pathologist to optimize vocal projec-

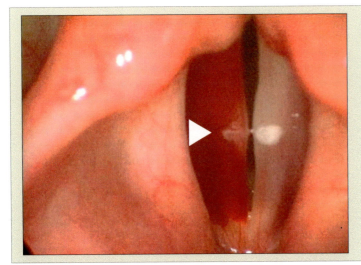

Figure 3–1. Right vocal fold hemorrhage (*arrowhead*).

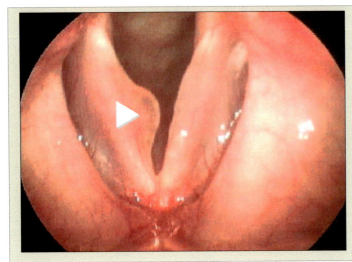

Figure 3–2. Right vocal fold polyp (*arrowhead*).

tion while eliminating strain can help to protect the voice and to prevent debilitating injury.

For those who use their voice for professional speaking, including acting and public speaking, as well as for singing, many of the same principles apply. In addition to routine vocal warm-ups and cool-downs at the start and end of the day, preparation (with exercises) for intense vocal use before vocal performance should routinely be employed.

Vocal Fold Lubrication

The vocal folds need adequate lubrication to maintain healthy vibration, particularly with prolonged phonation. This is achieved best by ensuring that the body is well hydrated at all times, but particularly prior to performing.

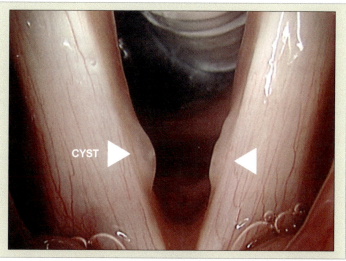

FIGURE 3–3. Right vocal fold cyst and left vocal fold reactive lesion (*arrowheads*).

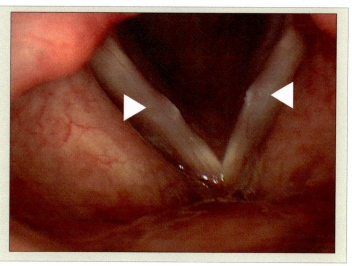

FIGURE 3–4. Bilateral vocal fold nodules (*arrowheads*).

Hydration is accomplished by drinking water or drinks that have balanced electrolytes, such as Gatorade™. Urine color is a good guide to the state of hydration. A pale urine color implies that there is adequate hydration for the kidneys, which usually is a good sign of adequate hydration throughout the body. Those with known kidney disorders, heart disease, hypertension, pituitary abnormalities, adrenal gland dysfunction, and other health problems should consult their physician and exercise caution before attempting to maintain hydration in this manner, as these individuals' usual mechanisms for fluid control may be impaired.

Water is preferred over juices or concentrated beverages. The sugar, salts, and sweeteners in such drinks limit the amount of water that is absorbed by the body. Caffeinated beverages and alcohol are dehydrating and should be avoided during and for several days prior to vocal performance (Table 3-1). It is most ideal for the busy voice to be hydrated at all times to prevent rapid changes in the body's fluid

TABLE 3–1. Foods and Beverages that Aggravate Reflux

- Dairy products (milk, cheese, yogurt, sour cream)
- Caffeine (coffee, tea, colas, chocolate)
- Acidic foods and beverages (tomatoes, oranges, pineapple juice)
- Fatty or fried foods (pizza, French fries, fried chicken)
- Processed meats (hot dogs, sausages, bratwursts)
- Spicy foods (including onions)
- Alcoholic beverages
- Peppermint
- Licorice

content. Because of the concern for reflux during performances, large quantities of liquid or water should not be consumed within the 2 hours prior to or during vocal performance.

MINIMIZING REFLUX

Because nearly everyone has some degree of reflux when intra-abdominal pressure is increased, care should be taken to minimize reflux episodes during vocal performance. Reflux is the regurgitation of stomach contents into the esophagus and occasionally larynx, throat, and/or nose and usually occurs when the pressure in the stomach surpasses that of the lower esophageal sphincter, the sling of muscles that is designed to help keep stomach contents in the stomach. For those utilizing proper breath support techniques for public speaking and singing, the abdominal pressures needed to project the voice can trigger a reflux episode.[4]

A common misconception is that reflux is synonymous with *heartburn*. Reflux episodes often occur without the sensation of heartburn. Heartburn is a symptom of severe and frequent refluxed gastric acid into the esophagus and is a sign of injury to the esophagus. Because the esophagus is lined by several layers of cells, it takes a significant amount of reflux to destroy these cells and cause deeper tissue injury. The larynx, portions of the throat, and nose are lined by tissue that is only one cell layer thick. It takes significantly less acid reflux to injure this cell layer and cause damage in the larynx and upper airway than it does to damage the lower esophagus.

Another way of understanding this concept is to use the skin on the back of the hand and the lining of the eye as analogies. Like the esophagus, the skin on the back of the hand is several cell layers thick, and like the larynx, the lining of the eye is only one cell layer thick. If one were to place a drop of vinegar (which is acidic) on the skin of the hand once daily, no visible damage would occur. If one were to place a drop of vinegar on the eye once daily, the eye would be chronically red, inflamed, and irritated. In this example, the drop of vinegar is analogous to occasional, mild reflux episodes, which typically do not cause heartburn or esophageal injury but frequently cause laryngeal injury and symptoms.

The stomach normally produces acid and enzymes to help digest food. If these reflux through the esophagus to the larynx, they may cause a contact irritation or laryngitis. Such irritation can trigger a cough, a sensation of tickle in the throat, the need for throat clearing, swelling of the vocal folds, a sensation of post-nasal drainage or phlegm in the throat, and they can alter the sensation (ability to feel) in the larynx.[5] These irritative behaviors can, in turn, result in vocal fold trauma and predispose to the formation of other vocal fold pathologies.

The best way to minimize reflux during vocal performance is to avoid eating meals or filling the stomach with liquids for at least 3 hours before performance, even in those who have no symptoms of reflux at all. Everyone has the potential to reflux when intra-abdominal pressure increases, especially the amount of abdominal pressure needed to support healthy phonation.

BREATH SUPPORT

Proper breath support is a key element of proper vocal technique in all forms of voice use and vocal performance. The lungs and related muscles of the chest, abdomen, and back are the power source for phonation and can be used to produce and modulate sound with minimal impact on the vocal folds themselves.

It is important when breathing to remember that the lungs are three-dimensional. Accordingly, expansion of the lungs should be both down into the abdomen and out on all sides. Inhalation should involve relaxation of the abdomen and back muscles, and exhalation should involve a sustained and controlled contraction of the abdominal and, perhaps to a lesser extent, the back muscles.

Phonation occurs during exhalation and should be supported by an adequate, inhaled breath prior to phonating. Proper posture with an erect spine, and with relaxation of the shoulders, muscles related to the collarbones, and shoulder blades, must be maintained.

RESONANCE

In addition to adequate breath support, proper positioning and alignment of the vocal tract aids in vocal projection and in minimizing trauma to the vocal folds. The positions of the tongue, jaw, larynx, and palate participate in the resonance of the voice as it leaves the larynx. Maximizing the effect of the resonator on the voice aids in vocal projection and minimizes the need for increased effort at the level of the vocal folds. The optimal position of each of these elements of the vocal tract varies depending upon the sound being produced, but in general, a more relaxed tongue, larynx, and jaw and an elevated palate produce a configuration of the vocal tract that helps to maximize vocal projection while minimizing vocal fold trauma.[6]

Baseline Laryngeal Evaluation

Early during one's career, every vocal performer should have a baseline laryngeal evaluation. The purpose of such an examination should be to evaluate the movement of the vocal folds and to diagnose any subtle abnormalities that may contribute to the development of vocal difficulties if left unattended.

The presence of mild vocal fold paresis is very common and is often thought of as the laryngeal equivalent of mildly poor vision.[7,8] Like mildly poor visual acuity, one can function reasonably well without correction; however, in some people, this problem can be debilitating and cause excess compensatory strain, especially in those who are not aware that they have the problem. Techniques as simple as vocal fold strengthening exercises and re-training of the involved muscles can help prevent the development of other pathologies in these individuals and can help improve vocal performance.[2,3]

Other subtle laryngeal abnormalities, such as reflux, that may have long-term effects on the voice can also be diagnosed and treated during a screening examination. Moreover, if asymptomatic abnormalities are present, it is important to be aware of them. Otherwise, if they are recognized first during a period of vocal problems, they may be diagnosed incorrectly as the cause of the complaint.

In some individuals, hoarseness and other vocal difficulties may develop as a result of illness. In these instances, it is useful to know if there were any preexisting pathologies and the relative contribution of these pathologies to the current vocal problem. Some individuals function well even in the presence of mild vocal fold weakness, small vocal fold polyps, nodules, or cysts and are unaware that these lesions exist unless they have had a baseline examination.[7] If a new vocal difficulty arises, particularly after an illness, it is helpful to know that these conditions were preexisting and likely not contributing significantly to the current vocal problem. Such knowledge can even help prevent the performance of unnecessary vocal fold surgery on benign lesions when vocal difficulties do arise.

Summary

Maintaining longevity of the voice involves attention to training and proper hygiene of the vocal folds throughout one's career. Daily stretching, attention to diet and hydration, and the use of proper vocal technique in all vocal situations are essential components of prolonged vocal health. Awareness of the health and state of one's larynx at baseline also can prove useful in preventing future problems and helpful in identifying the cause of new problems as they arise.

References

1. Sataloff RT. The human voice. *Scientific American* 1992; 267 (6): 108–115.
2. Sataloff RT. Structural abnormalities of the larynx. In: Sataloff RT. *Professional Voice: The Science and Art of Clinical Care*, 3rd ed. San Diego: Plural Publications; 2005: pp1255–1290.
3. Heuer RJ, Rulnick, Horman M, Perez KS, Emerich KA, Sataloff RT. Voice therapy. In: Sataloff RT. *Professional Voice: The Science and Art of Clinical Care*, 3rd ed. San Diego: Plural Publications; 2005: pp961–986.
4. Sataloff RT, Castell DO, Katz PO, Sataloff DM, Hawkshaw MJ. Reflux and other gastroenterologic conditions that may affect the voice. In: Sataloff RT. *Professional Voice: The Science and Art of*

Clinical Care, 3rd ed. San Diego: Plural Publications; 2005: pp591–652.
5. Koufman JA, Wiener GJ, Wu WC, Castell DO. Reflux laryngitis and its sequelae: the diagnostic role of ambulatory 24-hour pH monitoring. *Journal of Voice* 1988; 2:78–89.
6. Sundberg J. Vocal tract resonance. In: Sataloff RT. *Professional Voice: The Science and Art of Clinical Care*, 3rd ed. San Diego: Plural Publications; 2005: pp275–292.
7. Heman-Ackah YD, Dean C, Sataloff RT. Strobovideolaryngoscopic findings in singing teachers. *Journal of Voice* 2002; 16(1):81–86.
8. Heman-Ackah YD, Batory M. Determining the cause of mild vocal fold hypomobility. *Journal of Voice* 2003; 17(4):579–588.

▲ How Do I Find a Doctor and Voice Care Team?

4

Optimal voice care is delivered by an interdisciplinary team consisting of physicians and nonphysicians. The physician may be an otolaryngologist, a specialist who practices all aspects of ear, nose, and throat medicine, or a laryngologist, an otolaryngologist who specializes in voice disorders. The physician commonly collaborates with other professionals such as speech-language pathologists, singing voice specialists, acting voice specialists, voice scientists, nurses, psychologists, and others who constitute the voice care team.

Under the best of circumstances, all of the members of the team have received special training, not just in the general aspects of their disciplines, but also additional training in care of the voice. Although even the best training does not guarantee clinical excellence, it does improve the probability that a practitioner will provide superior, state-of-the-art voice care. This chapter reviews the typical training and qualifications of the professionals associated most commonly with voice care teams.

What Is a Voice Team?

A voice team is ordinarily under the direction of a physician who is usually an otolaryngologist or a laryngologist. In addition to the physician, the team also may include the following:

- speech-language pathologist
- phoniatrist (in countries without speech-language pathologist)
- singing voice specialist
- acting voice specialist
- voice scientist
- psychological professionals
- nurse and/or physician's assistant, and
- consultant physicians in other medical subspecialties.

The physician diagnoses and provides medical treatment for voice disorders. In some cases, the nurse and/or physician's assistant may assist the physician in patient care management. The physician may recommend voice therapy to correct functional, structural, and/or neurologic voice problems. Voice therapy is performed traditionally by the speech-language pathologist, but in some cases, training provided by a singing or acting voice specialist may be employed as well. When known or suspected medical conditions are contributing to an individual's voice disorder, referral to endocrinologists, rheumatologists, pulmonologists, gastroenterologists, general surgeons, psychiatrists, psychologists, neurologists, or other health professionals may be needed.

It is helpful for individuals who are seeking voice care to understand the background and role of each member of the voice team.

Who Are the Members of the Voice Team?

WHAT IS A LARYNGOLOGIST?

Laryngologists are otolaryngologists who specialize in care of disorders of the larynx and voice; in some cases, they also specialize in related problems such as swallowing and airway disorders.

To practice laryngology, one must first complete training as an otolaryngologist. After graduation from 4 years of medical school, otolaryngologists begin 1 year of training in general surgery and then 4 years of residency in otolaryngology–head and neck surgery. Following residency, the physician becomes a "board-eligible" otolaryngologist, a classification which indicates that the physician has met the minimum requirements needed to take the U.S. national board examinations.

Following successful completion of the board examination, the physician receives certification by the American Board of Otolaryngology. Becoming "board certified" by the American Board of Otolaryngology, or the American Board of Osteopathic Otolaryngology, or the equivalent organizations in other countries is an important indicator of mastery of basic knowledge in otolaryngology and is considered a basic, minimum credential.

Most otolaryngologists' clinical practices include many or all components of the specialty, such as:

- otology (the treatment of disorders of the ear)
- neurotology (treatment of the nerve connections between the ear and brain)
- laryngology (treatment of voice and airway disorders)
- head and neck surgery (the treatment of cancers and tumors in the head and neck)
- skull base surgery (treatment of cancers and tumors at the base of the skull and brain)
- facial plastic and reconstructive surgery
- rhinology (the treatment of nose, sinus, taste, and smell disorders)
- allergy and immunology (the treatment of allergy and problems with the

immune system)
- bronchoesophagology (lower airway and swallowing disorders), and
- pediatric otolaryngology (the treatment of otolaryngologic problems in children).

Most otolaryngologists and laryngologists care for patients of all ages, from early childhood through advanced years. Some subspecialize, caring for disorders in just one or two areas of otolaryngology as described above. This subspecialization can be either a keen interest in a specific area while still providing a broad range of otolaryngology care or a focused practice of only one or two of the subcomponents of otolaryngology. Laryngology is one such subspecialty.

Most otolaryngologists who subspecialize in one area complete a 1- or 2-year fellowship in that area before beginning the subspecialty practice. The fellowship is additional, focused training in a specific area of subspecialty, and completion of a fellowship usually implies a greater degree of competency and knowledge in that subspecialty than would be expected from a general otolaryngologist. Currently, within the specialty of otolaryngology, there exist recognized fellowships in laryngology, pediatric otolaryngology, facial plastic and reconstructive surgery, otology, neurotology, skull base surgery, head and neck surgery, allergy, and rhinology.

The practice of *voice care* is still considered to be in its "infancy," having been recognized only for a little more than three decades. At the present time, many physicians specializing in laryngology/voice care did not receive laryngology/voice fellowship training. That is always the case as a new field develops. Modern laryngology and voice care evolved out of an interest in caring for professional voice users, especially singers. The first comprehensive article guiding otolaryngologists on the care of professional singers was published in 1981.[1] The first major modern American otolaryngology textbook with a chapter on care of the professional voice was published in 1986.[2] The first comprehensive book on care of the professional voice was published in 1991.[3] Thus, most of the senior laryngologists practicing at the turn of the 21st century were involved in the evolution of the field, before fellowships were developed.

Fellowship training programs in laryngology and voice care started in the 1990s, although a few informal fellowship programs existed in the 1980s and earlier. It is reasonable to expect most voice specialists who finished residency training in the 1990s or later to have completed a fellowship in laryngology.

Currently, there are approximately 30 laryngology fellowship training programs in the United States, and they are highly competitive. Completion of a fellowship is a reasonably good indicator of superior knowledge and clinical training in laryngology. Most laryngology fellowships include training in the diagnosis, medical management, and surgical treatment of voice disorders, neurolaryngologic disorders (neurological problems that affect the voice and larynx), swallowing disorders, airway disorders, and laryngeal tumors and cancers in adults and children.

Laryngologists provide a wide spectrum of care for both routine and complex problems that affect the voice. Such problems include voice dysfunction associated with something as simple as a common cold (including acute laryngitis), especially when it affects the voice of a professional singer or actor. Laryngologists are responsible for the diagnosis and treatment of structural lesions such as nodules or polyps, prolonged infections of the vocal folds, cancer, traumatic injury from fracture or internal trauma (intubation injuries from anesthesia, vocal fold injuries from previous surgery), neurological disorders, and other voice problems. The laryngologist is responsible for establishing a medical diagnosis and implementing or coordinating treatment for the patient. Treatment may include prescription of medications, voice therapy, botulinum toxin injections, delicate microsurgery on the vocal folds, or operating through the neck on the laryngeal skeleton. Laryngologists are usually responsible for initiating evaluation by other members of the voice team and for generating referrals to other specialists as needed.

Laryngologists may practice in university medical centers or in private practice. In most cities in the United States, they are usually affiliated with a voice team. Laryngologists also should have, or have access to, a clinical voice laboratory with equipment to analyze the voice objectively and a stroboscope to visualize the vocal folds in slow motion. They also should be familiar with physicians in other specialties who have an understanding of and interest in arts medicine.[4] Even for patients with a voice disorder who are not singers and actors, such knowledge and sensitivity are important. Just as non-athletes benefit from the orthopedic expertise of a sports medicine specialist, voice patients receive more expert care from physicians trained to treat singers and actors, the "Olympic" athletes of the voice world.

At present, there is no official additional certification for those who have completed a laryngology fellowship. However, there are organizations (medical societies) with which many of the leading laryngologists are affiliated (Table 4-1). Essentially all laryngologists in the United States are fellows of the **American Academy of Otolaryngology–Head and Neck Surgery** (AAO-HNS), and laryngologists in other countries are members of their individual nation's analogous organizations. Additionally, it should be noted that some laryngologists outside the United States are associate members of the AAO-HNS.

A few are also members of the **American Laryngological Association** (ALA), the most senior otolaryngology society in the United States, which is limited to 150 active members. The ALA includes members who practice any or all areas of laryngology. Voice care may not be the area of interest for every member of the ALA. A physician must practice laryngology after completion of training for at least 7 years before becoming eligible for membership in the ALA, and many fellowship-trained laryngologists are not yet eligible to be members. The ALA also accepts associate members from other countries.

Some laryngologists belong to the **American Bronchoesophagological Association** (ABEA) and/or the Voice Foundation. The ABEA is an excellent professional organization that accepts many more members than the ALA, and at much less senior career status. Most ALA members also belong to the ABEA.

The Voice Foundation was founded in 1969 and is the oldest organization in the world dedicated solely to voice education and research. It provides seed grants for research, sponsors an annual symposium on care of the professional voice, and fosters voice education through conferences, educational videotapes, books, and publications such as the *Journal of Voice* and the *Voice Foundation Newsletter*.

In recent years, several countries have developed organizations similar to the Voice Foundation, such as the British, Canadian, and Australian Voice Founda-

TABLE 4–1. Selected List of Professional Organizations for Voice Team Members

Otolaryngologists/laryngologists
    American Academy of Otolaryngology–Head and Neck Surgery (AAO-HNS)   www.entnet.org
    American Laryngological Association (ALA)   www.alahns.org
    American Bronchoesophagological Association (ABEA)   www.abea.net
    The Voice Foundation   www.voicefoundation.org

Speech-language pathologists
    American Speech-Language-Hearing Association (ASHA)   www.asha.org

Singing voice specialists
    National Association of Teachers of Singing (NATS)   www.nats.org

Acting voice specialists
    Voice and Speech Trainers Association (VASTA)   www.vasta.org

Nurses
    Society of Otolaryngology-Head and Neck Nurses (SOHN)   www.sohnnurse.org

tions. Laryngologists in these countries are usually members of their national organizations, and many are also members of the Voice Foundation. While membership in these organizations is not a guarantee of excellence in practice, it suggests interest and knowledge in laryngology, particularly voice disorders.

WHAT IS A SPEECH-LANGUAGE PATHOLOGIST?

The speech-language pathologist (SLP) is a certified, licensed healthcare professional, ordinarily with either a Master's or PhD degree. After obtaining an undergraduate Bachelor's degree, speech-language pathologists generally complete a 1- or 2-year Master's degree program, followed by a 9-month, supervised clinical fellowship, similar to a medical internship. At the conclusion of the clinical fellowship year, SLPs in the United States are certified by the **American Speech-Language-Hearing Association** (ASHA) and use the letters CCC-SLP after their names to indicate that they are certified.

Like otolaryngology, speech-language pathology is a broad field that includes care of patients who have had strokes or other neurological problems affecting speech and swallowing, have undergone laryngectomy (removal of the larynx), have swallowing disorders, have articulation problems, stutter, have craniofacial disorders, or have other related fluency disorders of speech. Some SLPs subspecialize in voice, which includes the care of voice disorders. Speech pathology is the treatment of disorders of articulation, fluency, and prosody. Voice pathology is the treatment of disorders of voice production that primarily affect the larynx and that are unrelated to speech patterns, per se. The speech-language pathologist affiliated with a voice team is usually such a subspecialist and may call him- or herself a "voice pathologist" or "voice therapist" rather than a speech-language pathologist (although voice pathologist and voice therapist are not yet terms recognized officially by the ASHA).

There are relatively few speech-language pathology training programs that provide extensive education in voice, and there are virtually no voice fellowships for speech-language pathologists. Many speech-language pathology training programs do not even require a single course dealing with professional voice disorders. Thus, one can not assume that all SLPs are trained or comfortable in caring for individuals with voice problems. Most acquire the subspecialty training they need through apprenticeships, extra courses, symposia, or by obtaining PhDs that include voice-related research.

Speech-language pathologists are responsible for voice therapy and rehabilitation of the voice that is analogous to physical therapy. The SLP analyzes voice use and teaches proper breath support, relaxation, and voice placement to optimize use of the voice during speaking. A variety of techniques is utilized to accomplish this goal. SLPs ordinarily do not work with the singing voice, although they are involved in the treatment of the speaking voices of singers. The care provided by SLPs and singing voice specialists should be complementary. Patients should be cautioned about this, and if they feel they are not receiving the same approaches toward voice rehabilitation, they should discuss this with their laryngologist.

Speech-language pathologists may be found in universities, private offices, or free-standing speech and hearing centers. In the United States, most are members of ASHA and its voice-related special interest division. Many SLPs with special interest in voice in the U.S. and elsewhere are also members of the Voice Foundation.

Like otolaryngologists, SLPs who subspecialize in voice care provide more incisive, state-of-the-art treatment for voice disorders than most general SLPs who care for patients with various problems encompassing their entire scope of practice. Consequently, it is worthwhile for patients with voice disorders to seek a subspecialist to improve the likelihood of a rapid, excellent treatment result. Referrals to SLPs specializing in voice are usually obtained through a laryngologist or an otolaryngologist, who evaluates the larynx, provides a medical diagnosis, and coordinates care with the SLP.

WHAT IS A PHONIATRIST?

Phoniatrists do not exist in the United States, but in many countries outside the U.S., they provide voice care. The phoniatrist is a physician who is in some ways a hybrid of the laryngologist and the speech-language pathologist. Phoniatrists receive medical training in diagnosis and treatment of voice, swallowing, and language disorders, including voice therapy, but they do not perform surgery. In countries with phoniatrists, surgery is performed by otolaryngologists. In many cases, the phoniatrist and otolaryngologist collaborate as a team, just as otolryngologists and speech-language pathologists do in the United States. A physician who has completed training in phoniatry is generally well qualified to diagnose voice disorders and provide nonsurgical medical care as well as voice therapy.

WHAT IS A SINGING VOICE SPECIALIST?

The singing voice specialist is a singing teacher with special training equipping him or her to practice in a medical environment with patients who have sustained vocal injury. Most singing voice specialists have a degree in voice performance or pedagogy, although some have only extensive performing and teaching experience without a formal academic degree. Nearly all have extra training in laryngeal anatomy and physiology of phonation, training in the rehabilitation of injured voices, and other special education.

The singing voice specialist must acquire knowledge of anatomy and physiology of the normal and disordered voice, a basic understanding of the principles of laryngology, medications used to treat voice disorders, medications and herbal remedies that can potentially harm the voice, and the principles and practices of speech-language pathology. This information is not part of the traditional training of singing teachers. Moreover, at present, there are no formal training or fellowship programs that assist singing teachers in becoming singing voice specialists. Their training is acquired by apprenticeship and observation.

Many take courses in speech-language pathology programs, but usually not as part of a formal degree or certification program, since there is still no certification of singing voice specialists.[5] A few of the best singing voice specialists are also certified, licensed speech-language pathologists. This combination is optimal, provided the speech-language pathologist has sufficient experience and training not only as a performing artist but also as a teacher of singing.

In patients with vocal injuries or problems, the fundamental approach to training the singing voice is different in important ways from that usually used with healthy students in a singing studio. Hence, even an excellent and experienced voice teacher may harm, rather than help, an injured voice, if he or she is not familiar with the special considerations for this population. In addition, a knowledgeable and enlightened singing teacher generally will not feel comfortable working with a singer who has had a vocal injury or surgery.

Virtually all singing voice specialists are affiliated with voice care teams. Most are members of the **National Association of Teachers of Singing** (NATS) or the equivalent organization in another country and of the Voice Foundation. In many cases, their practices are limited to work with injured voices. They work not only with singers, but also with other patients with voice disorders. As members of a voice treatment team working with nonsingers, they help teach speakers the "athletic" techniques utilized by singers for voice production. Singing is to speaking as running is to walking. When rehabilitating someone who has difficulty walking, if the person can be helped to jog or run, leg strength and endurance improve and walking rehabilitation is expedited. The singing voice specialist helps apply similar principles to voice rehabilitation, in collaboration with the speech-language pathologist and other voice care team members.

WHAT IS AN ACTING VOICE SPECIALIST?

Acting voice specialists/trainers are also called *voice coaches, drama voice teachers,* and *voice consultants.* Traditionally, these professionals have been associated closely with the theater. Their skills have been utilized as part of a medical voice team only since the mid 1990s.[6] Consequently, there are few acting voice trainers with medical experience, but their contributions have proven to be invaluable.

Acting voice trainers use a variety of behavior modification techniques that have been designed to enhance vocal communication, quality, projection, and endurance in theatrical settings. They train actors to speak or scream through eight shows a week, or perhaps through theatrical runs that may last years, without tiring or causing injury to their voices. They also teach techniques for adding emotional expression to vocal delivery, and they work with body language and posture to optimize vocal delivery and communication of information.

They can be a great asset to the voice team in teaching people how to apply the many skills learned through the speech-language pathologist and singing voice specialist to their everyday life. Acting voice trainers are especially valuable for people who speak professionally, such as lawyers, teachers, lecturers, politicians, clergy, sales personnel, and others concerned with effective vocal delivery and with vocal endurance.

There are no formal programs that prepare voice coaches to work in a medical milieu. Those who do work in medical centers receive training through apprenticeships and collaborations with medical voice care teams, under the direction of a laryngologist. Acting voice trainers interested in working with voice patients are generally members of the **Voice and Speech Trainers Association** (VASTA) and the Voice Foundation.

WHAT IS THE ROLE OF THE VOICE SCIENTIST?

Voice scientists are typically speech-language pathologists or voice specialists with an advanced degree who have a special interest in the science and physiology (physical mechanism) of normal and disordered voice production. However, an increasing number of specialists in other disciplines have also become voice scientists, including physicists, engineers, and others. Voice scientists measure a myriad of parameters that reflect lung function, lung capacity, breath support, vocal fold closure patterns, and clarity of the voice. The measurements obtained by the voice scientist help to guide voice therapy and medical decisions, particularly decisions pertaining to the role of surgery, in the treatment of voice difficulties.

WHAT IS THE ROLE OF NURSES ON THE VOICE TEAM?

Nurses are an indispensable asset in medical offices, and they are important members of the voice team in many centers. Nurses who work closely with a laryngologist generally have vast experience in the diagnosis and treatment of voice disorders. They are wonderful informational resources for patients and frequently provide much of the patient education in busy clinical settings. Such nurses are usually members of the **Society of Otolaryngology-Head and Neck Nurses** (SOHN). Nurses with advanced knowledge and skills may be certified by SOHN and are identified as such by the initials CORLN, (certified otorhinolaryngologic nurse), after their names.

Nurse practitioners are advanced practice nurses with Master's degrees who are licensed to provide independent care for patients with selected medical problems. They are identified by the initials CRNP (certified registered nurse practitioner). They work in conjunction with a physician, but they can examine, diagnose, and treat selected problems relatively independently. A few nurse practitioners specialize in otolaryngology and work with voice teams. They ordinarily receive special "on the job" training by the otolaryngologist, and they provide care within their scope of practice. Nurse practitioners can also become members of SOHN, become certified through examination by SOHN, and upon certification will also use the initials CORLN after their names.

What Are Physician Assistants and Medical Assistants?

Physician assistants, like nurse practitioners, function in association with a physician. Physician assistants graduate from a 4-year training program that teaches them various aspects of medical diagnosis and physical examination. They use the initials PAC (physician assistant-certified) after their names.

Physician assistants practice in conjunction with physicians, but can perform examinations and treat patients independently. They are licensed in many states to write prescriptions. Some physician assistants specialize in otolaryngology and even a smaller number subspecialize in laryngology, which requires extensive training and experience in voice care. In collaboration with a laryngologist and voice teams, they are qualified to evaluate and treat patients with voice disorders.

Physician assistants are distinctly different from medical assistants, who have less training and are qualified to assist in medical care and patient education, but cannot diagnose or treat patients independently. Medical assistants generally are trained to perform tasks such as phlebotomy (drawing blood) and obtaining electrocardiograms. In a laryngology office, a good medical assistant can be trained to perform many other tasks, such as taking histories, assisting with strobovideolaryngoscopy, assisting during the performance of surgical procedures in the office, participating in research, and other similar duties.

What Medical Consultants Are Associated with the Voice Team?

Otolaryngologists often refer voice patients for consultation with other medical professionals. Specialists who are consulted commonly include neurologists, pulmonologists, gastroenterologists, psychologists, psychiatrists, and general surgeons. However, physicians in virtually any medical specialty may be called upon to care for voice patients. Traditional and nontraditional ancillary medical personnel also may be involved in voice care, including nutritionists, physical therapists, chiropractors, osteopathic physicians specializing in manipulation, acupuncturists, and others.

Within virtually all these fields, there are a select number of physicians and professionals who have an interest in and an understanding of arts medicine, including care of the professional voice. Many such physicians tend to be associated with arts medicine centers or are performers themselves. There is no certification board, national or international organization that helps to identify such physicians, although some are members of the **Performing Arts Medicine Association** (PAMA) in the United States or similar groups internationally (Table 4-2). In most fields, there are no formal arts medicine training programs or associations.

Physicians acquire such training through their own interests and initiative and through apprenticeship or observation with colleagues.

If there is no arts medicine center in the area in which an individual is seeking care, arts medicine physicians are identified best by word of mouth or through arts medicine-related websites. Referrals can be obtained through the local laryngologist or voice specialist or by consulting with prominent performing arts teachers in the community. For example, the leading private, university, and conservatory violin and piano teachers often know who the best hand specialists are, and the same is true for other instrumental music or dance teachers.

When Should I Seek Out an Laryngologist Instead of a General Otolaryngologist?

Most otolaryngologists possess basic familiarity with common voice disorders that affect most people in the population, such as laryngitis during an upper respiratory tract infection (the common "cold"). However, management of even simple problems such as laryngitis is different in professional voice users. People with special voice needs may be served best by consulting a laryngologist with a special interest or concentration in voice disorders, even for common problems. Laryngologists also are helpful in more complex problems that may be difficult for general otolaryngologists to diagnose or treat since general otolaryngologists do not see unusual voice disorders on a daily basis and also may not have essential diagnostic equipment such as a stroboscope. If a patient has seen an otolaryngologist a few times for voice problems and is not getting better, obtaining an opinion from a physician subspecializing in laryngology may be most helpful, especially if the cause of the voice problem has not been identified with certainty.

Consultation with a laryngologist also should be considered when surgery is recommended, particularly surgery for benign problems such as nodules, cysts, and polyps. The technology and standard of care for voice microsurgery has changed dramatically over the last 10 to 15 years. Laryngologists should be familiar with state-of-the-art treatment in voice care, but it is impossible for general otolaryngologists to be up to date in every aspect of ear, nose, and throat care.

ARE THERE ANY "RED FLAGS" THAT SHOULD MAKE ME GET A SECOND OPINION IMMEDIATELY?

Yes! If a physician recommends immediate "emergency" surgery for benign problems such as nodules, a second opinion should be obtained. There are very few indications for "emergency" voice surgery.

Most surgical procedures to improve the voice should also include voice therapy as part of the treatment regimen. If voice therapy is not recommended both before and after removal of a benign vocal fold mass, a second opinion should be sought, as the lack of such a recommendation implies (in most cases) an insufficient understanding of the treatment of voice disorders.

TABLE 4–2. Selected List of Performing Arts Medicine Associations Worldwide

- Performing Arts Medicine Association (PAMA) (USA) — www.artsmed.org
- American Alliance for Health, Physical Education, Recreation and Dance (AAHPERD) (USA) — www.aahperd.org/aahperd/
- APTA Performing Arts Special Interest Group (USA) (associated with American Physical Therapy Assoc.) — www.orthopt.org/sig_pa.php
- Artists' Health Centre Foundation (Canada) — www.ahcf.ca/
- Arts Medicine Aotearoa NZ (New Zealand) — www.converge.org.nz/amanz/
- Australian Dance Council — www.ausdance.org.au/
- Australian Society for Performing Arts Healthcare — www.aspah.org.au
- British Association for Performing Arts Medicine — www.bapam.org.uk/
- Deutsche Gesellschaft fur Musikphysiologie and Musikermedizin (German Association for Music Physiology and Musicians' Medicine) — www.dgfmm.org/
- Finnish Society for Musician's Medicine (SMULY)
- International Association for Dance Medicine and Science — www.iadms.org/
- Medecine des Arts (France) — www.medecine-des-arts.com
- Nederlandse Vereniging voor Dans- en MuziekGeneeskunde (NVDMG) (Dutch Performing Arts Medicine Association) — www.nvdmg.org
- Österreichische Gesellschaft für Musik und Medizin (OGfMM) (Austrian Society for Music and Medicine) — www.oegfmm.at/
- Schweizerische Gesellschaft für Musik-Medizin (Swiss Association for Music-Medicine) — www.musik-medizin.ch
- TanzMedizin Deutschland (German Dance Medicine Association) — www.tamed.de
- The Voice Foundation (USA) — www.voicefoundation.org

In addition, if the physician uses the words "vocal fold stripping," it implies an antiquated surgical technique that is more likely to result in permanent hoarseness than more delicate phonomicrosurgical approaches. If stripping is recommended, a second opinion should be sought from an expert laryngologist.

How Do I Find an Expert Laryngologist?

Guidelines for finding an expert laryngologist are discussed earlier in the section on laryngologists. Contacting organizations such as the Voice Foundation or the American Laryngological Association is a good start. It is also reasonable to check the literature and the Internet to see who has written articles or books about voice problems like the one for which a patient is seeking care.

Because most laryngologists are affiliated with major academic medical centers, those who do not live near such centers may need to travel several hundred miles to find a qualified laryngologist. For most, the level of care given by those who subspecialize in laryngology and professional voice care is well worth the time and cost spent in traveling

Do I Really Need to See Other (Nonphysician) Members of the Voice Team?

Most of the time, the entire voice team plays an integral role in the diagnosis of the voice problem and in the rehabilitation of the voice, and it is important for patients to follow through on all aspects of therapy.

The *speech-language pathologist* is invaluable in diagnosing and correcting errors in voice usage that can cause or aggravate voice dysfunction. In nearly all cases, patients use hyperfunctional voicing in an attempt to compensate for their voice disorders. It is always important to eliminate the hyperfunction to unmask the true nature of the voice disorders. Moreover, in many cases, voice therapy alone is enough to cure the problem. For example, more than 90% of vocal fold nodules resolve or become asymptomatic through voice therapy, without surgery.

The *singing voice specialist* not only defines and rectifies similar inefficient muscle use patterns in singers, but also teaches nonsingers some of the athletic exercises and tricks used by singers to improve vocal control, volume, projection, quality, and variability. Even in someone with no skill or interest in singing, these athletic techniques can be applied to the speaking voice quickly and can speed vocal recovery.

The *acting voice specialist* helps integrate optimal techniques into daily use and teaches additional methods for improving vocal expression and the overall impact of personal communication. Learning the techniques used by actors to project a message efficiently allows all voice users to get their points across skillfully, without vocal strain

Is It Safe to Be Seen at a Teaching Hospital or Clinic?

Virtually all of the leading voice specialists and voice care teams are affiliated with medical schools and teaching hospitals. Most laryngologists will examine, treat, and perform surgery on their patients themselves, sometimes with the assistance of residents and/or laryngology fellows.

Residents are physicians who have already completed college, 4 years of medical school, 1 year of general surgery training, are completing their training in otolaryngology (a 4-year training period itself). The residents are always supervised by the otolaryngologist or laryngologist, who is primarily responsible for the care of the patient. The laryngology *fellow* has completed his/her residency in otolaryngology and is board eligible and, in some cases, is board certified. The fellow also works under the supervision of the laryngologist. In some cases, medical students may also be involved in the care of the patients, but they are not responsible for hands-on care as would be the resident or fellow.

The teaching environment encourages the most advanced state-of-the-art care, and most cutting-edge technologies are found in academic medical centers. Although information usually is kept about treatment outcomes as part of the process of self-critique, through which clinical care is improved, being seen at a teaching hospital does not mean that you are going to be part of an experiment. Any procedures or protocols that are experimental are identified clearly, and patients are always given the option of participating or not participating. Often, these experimental opportunities represent the best, cutting-edge therapy for problems that are generally considered untreatable. Such experimental, advanced treatment is usually made available only by physicians who are affiliated with teaching programs and are always kept confidential.

If I Find the Best Laryngologist and the Best Voice Team, Am I Guaranteed a Good Result?

No. Even if everything is done perfectly, sometimes outcomes are disappointing. In most cases, bad outcomes, such as permanent hoarseness from scarring after vocal fold surgery, are due to healing problems that are neither the fault of the physician nor the voice team nor the patient. As an analogy, if a surgeon makes a similar appendectomy incision on 100 consecutive patients, a few of them may develop a large or wide scar, even though the incision was made and sutured perfectly each time.

There are uncertainties involved with the human body, and even the best care in the world does not guarantee a perfect outcome. However, it does decrease the chance of a bad outcome. Optimal results require the best efforts of every member of the voice care team, including the patient, who is the most important member of the team. Compliance with voice therapy, medical therapy, anti-reflux measures, good technical voice use, and voice rest, when prescribed, are essential to "stack the odds" in favor of an optimal result.

Summary

Voice care has evolved into a sophisticated, well-organized medical science. Patients with voice disorders are served best by a comprehensive voice team that coordinates the skills of professionals trained in various disciplines. The team usually includes a laryngologist or otolaryngologist as its leader, but also other professionals such as a speech-language pathologist, a singing or acting voice specialist, a psychologist, and a nurse or physician assistant. It is important for health care professionals to assemble interdisciplinary teams and to affiliate with arts medicine specialists and other disciplines to provide comprehensive care for voice patients. It is also important for patients to be educated about the kind of health care that is now available for voice disorders and how to evaluate and select health care providers.

References

1. Sataloff RT. Professional singers: the science and art of clinical care. *American Journal of Otolaryngology* 1981; 2(3):251–266.
2. Sataloff RT. The professional voice. In: Cummings CW, Frederickson JM, Harker LA, Krause CJ, Schuller DE, eds. *Otolaryngology–Head and Neck Surgery*. St. Louis: CV Mosby; 1986: pp2029–2056.
3. Sataloff RT. *Professional Voice: The Science and Art of Clinical Care*. New York: Raven Press; 1991.
4. Sataloff RT, Brandfonbrenner A, Lederman R, eds. *Performing Arts Medicine*, 2nd ed. San Diego: Singular Publishing Group, Inc.; 1998.
5. Sataloff RT, Baroody MM, Emerich KA, Carroll LM, Sataloff RT. The singing voice specialist. In: Sataloff RT. *Professional Voice: The Science and Art of Clinical Care*, 3rd ed. San Diego: Plural Publications; 2005: pp1021–1040.
6. Freed SL, Raphael BN, Sataloff RT. The role of the acting voice trainer in medical care of professional voice users. In: Sataloff RT. *Professional Voice: The Science and Art of Clinical Care*, 3rd ed. San Diego: Plural Publications; 2005: pp1051–1060.

5

▲ When Should I See a Voice Doctor?

C are of the voice involves two main aspects: prevention and treatment of acute and chronic voice disorders. These are the two reasons to see a voice doctor.

Preventative Voice Care

Anyone who relies on his or her voice professionally should have a baseline laryngeal function and videostroboscopic examination with a laryngologist when the voice is functioning optimally and without difficulty. This examination will help to diagnose any potential areas of concern that may contribute, in the long term, to the development of debilitating voice difficulties. Entities such as asymptomatic reflux, mild asymmetries in vocal fold motion, allergy, tonsil enlargement, nasal septal deviation, nasal congestion, nasal polyps, and others that may not be causing any difficulties presently, but may contribute to the development of voice problems in the future, can be identified and recommendations can be made by the laryngologist and voice team on how to prevent these entities from becoming problematic. Additionally, asymptomatic benign lesions, such as polyps, cysts, pseudocysts (localized swelling in the vocal fold), areas of stiffness, sulcus vocalis (benign indentations in the vocal fold), and others, can be identified.

Knowing that these lesions exist when the voice is functioning normally can prevent a misdiagnosis and misguided treatment that may otherwise focus on these lesions as the cause of a voice problem in the future. Because everyone is at risk for infection, trauma, and the need for non-voice surgery that may require general anesthesia, everyone is at risk for the development of voice problems, regardless of one's level of training, technical prowess, or use of proper voice technique.

Upper respiratory infection (colds) may predispose a person to vocal injury, especially if the illness includes hoarseness. Care should be taken to avoid heavy

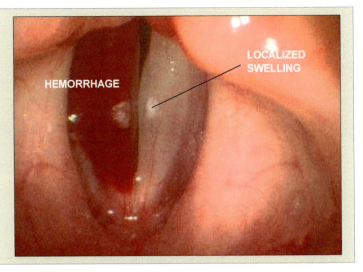

FIGURE 5–1. Right vocal fold hemorrhage, with localized swelling (pseudocyst) of the left vocal fold.

voice use during a cold and to avoid taking cold medications that contain blood thinners (such as aspirin and ibuprofen), which may cause vocal fold hemorrhage. If hoarseness persists after a cold has resolved, a laryngologist should be consulted.

SUDDEN HOARSENESS

Probably the most pressing reason to see a voice clinician is to evaluate acute voice disorders that may worsen if left untreated. These usually are characterized by the sudden onset of hoarseness and can be precipitated by a myriad of events, including trauma, voice overuse or misuse, and infection.

The sudden onset of hoarseness during or immediately after intense vocal use implies injury to the vocal fold. This may be in the form of hemorrhage, tear, or edema.

- Hemorrhage (Figure 5-1) occurs when there is trauma to one of the blood vessels within the vocal fold and it begins to bleed. Usually the bleeding is beneath the surface of the vocal fold mucosal cover, and the only symptom of the bleeding is the occurrence of hoarseness and occasionally soreness or pain in the throat.[1]
- A vocal fold tear occurs when there is disruption of the mucous membrane of the vocal fold, usually from intense yelling, screaming, or forceful singing.[1] Vocal fold tears can also occur during episodes of laryngitis or other upper respiratory tract or gastrointestinal infections, usually as a result of coughing forcefully, from dry heaves, or from wretching during vomiting. The placement of an endotracheal (breathing) tube by an anesthesiologist for surgery can also result in vocal fold tears (Figure 5-2).
- Edema (Figure 5-3) is swelling in response to vocal fold trauma or infection.

Each of these entities represents a vocal emergency and should be evaluated immediately, especially if the hoarseness began abruptly enough to interrupt the

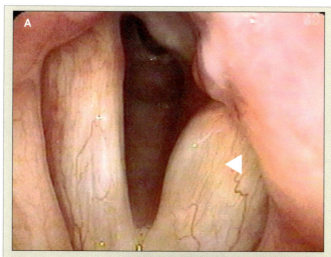
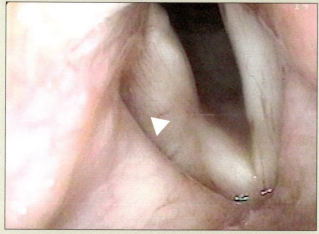

FIGURE 5–2. A, Left vocal fold shortening and scarring (*arrow*) with subglottic stenosis following intubation injury. **B,** Scarring of the right mid-vocal fold (*arrow*) following laceration of the vocal fold from intubation.

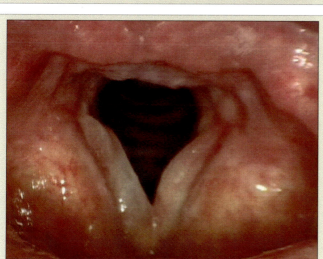

FIGURE 5–3. Bilateral vocal fold edema.

conclusion of a sentence, phrase, or performance, or immediately following surgery or a coughing/vomiting episode.

The treatment of vocal fold hemorrhage varies depending upon the degree of bleeding. In most instances, a period of absolute voice rest is all that is needed. On occasion, the hemorrhage is significant enough to warrant immediate surgical drainage. In these cases, if left alone, the hemorrhage may organize to form a polyp and/or, potentially, scarring of the vocal fold.

Vocal fold tears are treated with a period of voice rest to allow the tear to heal. If the tear is superficial, usually healing will occur without significant sequelae if the voice is rested. If the tear is deep, there is greater potential for scarring, which can have more significant long-term implications. In either case, if one continues to phonate on a vocal fold that is torn, the risk of permanent scarring appears to increase. Once scarring of the vocal fold has formed, it is difficult to treat and often results in permanent hoarseness and/or difficulty with register transitions.

Edema of the vocal fold occurs from several causes, including phonotrauma from forceful closure of the vocal folds. This can occur in an individual who is yelling or screaming, in one who is trying to talk or sing with an upper respiratory tract infection, as well as in those who are trying to project the voice by increasing pressure in the vocal folds. Edema alone usually resolves with a period of relative voice rest or light voice use. Relative voice rest is near complete silence, reserving the voice for urgent communication only. Light voice use is minimal talking, usually no more than about 5 minutes per hour and no more than approximately 1 minute continuously at a time.

On occasion, corticosteroids can be used to speed recovery from vocal fold edema, but they should be used cautiously. Typically, steroids cause one to feel and sound much better than the actual health of the vocal folds and can predispose to further vocal fold trauma if attention to good vocal technique is not employed while using these medications.

NECK TRAUMA

External trauma to the neck can result in injury to the larynx and requires urgent evaluation by a doctor. Such trauma can occur from incidents such as elbowing to the neck while playing basketball or during a stage fight, from automobile accidents in which the neck hits the steering wheel or is caught by the safety belt, the falling of the neck onto the handlebars of a bicycle, or strangulation or choking injuries to the neck.

Injuries from blunt neck trauma can include nerve paresis (weakness), cartilage fracture, joint dislocation, and vocal fold hemorrhage, edema, or tear.[2] These injuries can be potentially life threatening, especially if the airway collapses suddenly from fracture or if swelling develops following the injury. Immediate medical attention is recommended in all cases, even if mild hoarseness is the only symptom. Many individuals who suffer a blunt neck injury feel fine initially, and swelling or a sudden shift in the fractured cartilages occurs minutes or hours after the trauma, obstructing the airway in a manner that can be life threatening.

During such injuries, the recurrent laryngeal nerve can become crushed between the spine and the cricoid cartilage, resulting in a nerve paresis. This typically manifests as hoarseness or breathiness in the voice. Vocal fatigue and effortful phonation are also symptoms. The treatment of vocal fold paresis from neck trauma is usually symptomatic (including voice therapy and occasionally surgery), and unless the nerve is severed, function will usually improve over the course of weeks to months.

Fracture of the laryngeal cartilages and dislocation of the cricothyroid and/or cricoarytenoid joints can also occur as a result of neck trauma. Symptoms of these injuries usually include hoarseness, pain, and occasionally difficulty breathing. Fracture or dislocation is a medical emergency and warrants evaluation by a laryngologist or otolaryngologist to determine whether the airway is at risk and whether surgical intervention is necessary. Even in the absence of airway compromise, the determination as to whether a fracture or dislocation should be corrected is best made within the first 24 to 48 hours after injury. During this time frame, attempts at reduction of the fractured or dislocated segments are easiest and are most likely to yield the best long-term results. If too much time is allowed to pass before treatment is initiated, scarring and healing of the fragments in abnormal locations may occur.[3-5]

HOARSENESS AFTER SURGERY

Hoarseness after a surgical procedure performed on an area outside the larynx warrants special mention. During general anesthesia for most surgical procedures, an endotracheal (breathing) tube is placed into the larynx, between the vocal folds, to help maintain respiration while the patient is asleep. Vocal fold trauma (mucosal tear or hemorrhage) can occur during the advancement of the tube into the larynx or upon removal of the tube when the patient is awakened from anesthesia.

Laryngeal trauma from intubation usually is managed with voice rest and is a well-recognized complication of anesthesia. Whenever possible, the smallest (5.0 to 6.0 mm inner diameter) plastic endotracheal tube that will allow adequate ventilation (artificial breathing) during general anesthesia is recommended for professional voice users undergoing non-voice surgery.

In some individuals, the placement of the endotracheal tube can result in injury to a vocal fold or even dislocation of the arytenoid cartilage from its position on the cricoid cartilage. This dislocation may happen occasionally with even the most skilled of anesthesiologists. Usually, the patient awakens from anesthesia with a hoarse voice that does not improve with time. Arytenoid dislocations are best treated as early as possible to prevent permanent scarring around the dislocated cartilage. If scar forms, reduction can become difficult. As soon as the diagnosis is suspected, consultation with an otolaryngologist should be made.[3-5]

Another cause of hoarseness after nonlaryngeal surgery is injury to the recurrent or superior laryngeal nerves. This may occur during any surgical procedure that is performed in the vicinity of the nerves in the neck or chest and occasionally after intubation for surgery outside the head and neck. Because the nerves travel a long route from the brain, into the neck and chest, and back through the neck to enter

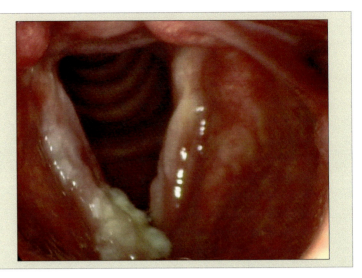

Figure 5-4. Right vocal fold cancer.

the larynx, injury may occur with surgery in any of these locations.[6] Like arytenoid dislocation, patients who experience injury to the laryngeal nerves during surgery usually awaken from surgery with a hoarse and/or breathy voice.

All patients who have hoarseness after non-voice surgery should have their larynx examined immediately by a laryngologist. Differentiation between an arytenoid dislocation and nerve injury can be difficult in these instances, and diagnosis usually is made with the aid of laryngeal examination, laryngeal electromyography, and computed tomography scanning.

The treatment of laryngeal nerve injury varies depending upon whether the nerve is suspected of having been cut or just stretched. A stretched, intact nerve usually will recover on its own over the course of weeks to months. Treatment in these instances is symptomatic and may include corticosteroids, collagen injection, gelfoam injection, fat injection, or thyroplasty to place the vocal fold in a favorable position for eating and speaking while it recovers. A nerve that is suspected of having been severed should be repaired as soon as the suspicion is raised to maximize the chances of maintaining good laryngeal tone.

PROLONGED HOARSENESS

Anyone who experiences hoarseness or another vocal difficulty that persists longer than 2 weeks should have his or her larynx evaluated by a laryngologist or otolaryngologist. It is rare for a "laryngitis" alone to persist for more than 2 weeks, even if the hoarseness began during an upper respiratory tract infection. In such instances, the persistent hoarseness may be due to a mild paresis of the vocal folds, which can occur when the virus that causes the upper respiratory tract infection infects the nerve, causing it to swell and weaken. Hoarseness that does not resolve following an upper respiratory tract infection should be evaluated.[7]

Alternatively, other pathologies in the larynx, including cancer (Figure 5-4) and human papilloma virus infections (Figure 5-5), may begin with a similar pres-

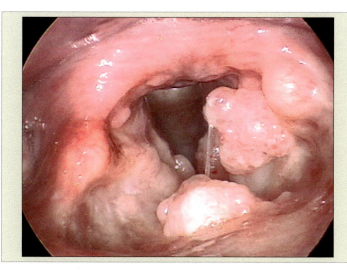

FIGURE 5–5. Laryngeal papillomas.

entation and should be evaluated. If left untreated, these lesions may grow large enough to obstruct the airway, limit breathing, and potentially cause death.

Summary

There are several instances in which the larynx should be evaluated promptly. These include hoarseness that is abrupt in onset, hoarseness that begins immediately after non-voice surgery, trauma to the larynx or neck, and hoarseness that persists for longer than 2 weeks, even if the onset was during the course of an upper respiratory tract infection. The reasons for evaluation in these instances are the prevention of long-term sequelae, such as permanent hoarseness, scarring, and vocal fold lesions, and the diagnosis and treatment of potentially life-threatening illnesses such as cancer, tumors, and airway compromise. Having a baseline laryngeal evaluation when vocal production is optimal is also advocated as a preventative health measure. Knowledge of one's unique anatomy in the "normal" state will help to guide diagnosis and treatment should voice difficulties later arise, whether they be from disease, infection, trauma, or abnormal use patterns.

References

1. Heman-Ackah YD, Sataloff RT. Blunt trauma to the larynx and trachea: considerations for the professional voice user. *Journal of Singing* 2002; 59(1):41–47.
2. Heman-Ackah YD, Goding GS Jr, Rao V. Laryngotracheal trauma. In: Rubin JS, Sataloff RT, Korovin GS, eds. *Diagnosis and Treatment of Voice Disorders*, 3rd ed. San Diego: Plural Publishing, Inc.; 2006.
3. Sataloff RT, Feldman M, Darby KS, Carroll LM, Spiegel JR. Arytenoid dislocation. *Journal of Voice*

1987; 1:368–377.
4. Sataloff RT, Bough ID, Spiegel JR. Arytenoid dislocation: diagnosis and treatment. *Laryngoscope* 1994; 104:1353–1361.
5. Sataloff RT. *Professional Voice: The Science and Art of Clinical Care*, 3rd ed. San Diego: Plural Publishing, Inc.; 2005.
6. Heman-Ackah YD, Batory M. Determining the cause of mild vocal fold hypomobility. *Journal of Voice* 2003; 17(4):579–588.
7. Dursun G, Sataloff RT, Spiegel JR, Mandel S, Heuer RJ, Rosen DC. Superior laryngeal nerve paresis and paralysis. *Journal of Voice* 1996; 10:206–211.

6
▲ What Can I Expect During a Visit to the Voice Doctor?

Until the 1980s, most physicians caring for patients with voice disorders asked only a few basic questions, such as: "How long have you been hoarse?," "Do you smoke?," etc. The physician's ear was the sole "instrument" used routinely to assess voice quality and function. Visualization of the vocal folds was limited to looking with a mirror placed inside the mouth using regular light or using direct laryngoscopy (looking directly at the vocal folds through a metal pipe or endoscope) under anesthesia in the operating room. Treatment was generally limited to medicines for infection or inflammation, surgery for bumps or masses, and no treatment if the vocal folds looked "normal." Occasionally, "voice therapy" was recommended, but the specific nature of therapy was not well controlled, and results were often disappointing. Since the early 1980s, the standard of care has changed dramatically

What Kinds of Questions Are Expected from One's Doctor?

Correct medical diagnosis in all fields often hinges on asking the right questions and then listening carefully to the answers. This process is known as "taking a history" and is usually the first step of the initial office visit encounter. The history may be taken directly by the physician or may be taken by a nurse or medical assistant, who then relates the history to the physician.

Recently, medical care for voice problems has utilized a markedly expanded, comprehensive history that recognizes that there is more to the voice than simply the vocal folds. Virtually any body system may be responsible for voice complaints. In fact, problems outside the larynx often cause voice dysfunction in people whose vocal folds appear fairly normal, and these issues need to be relayed to the physician and/or the medical staff at the time of the history.

Regardless of whether or not the patient feels that portions of their medical or surgical history, including the use of medications, herbal remedies, or vitamin supplements are relevant to their voice problem, it is extremely important that the voice doctor and the voice team are aware of everything that is currently affecting, or in the past has affected, the function of the entire body.

DESCRIBE YOUR HOARSENESS

The first question asked in the office encounter is for the individual to describe, in detail, the difficulties that he or she is having with his or her voice. Most people with voice problems complain of "hoarseness" or "laryngitis." A more accurate description of the problem is often helpful in identifying the cause, and the laryngologist will usually ask several questions to help gain a better understanding the voice problem and its possible causes.

Hoarseness can be described as *raspiness*, which is a coarse, scratchy sound caused most commonly by abnormalities on the vibratory margin of the vocal fold. These may include swelling, roughness from inflammation, growths, scarring, or anything that interferes with vocal fold vibration. Such abnormalities produce turbulence at the level of the glottis, which is perceived as raspiness.

Breathiness is caused by lesions (abnormalities) that keep the vocal folds from closing completely, including paresis (partial weakness), paralysis (complete weakness), cricoarytenoid joint injury or arthritis, vocal fold masses, scarring, or atrophy (wasting) of the vocal fold tissues. These abnormalities permit air to escape when the vocal folds are supposed to be tightly closed. We hear this air leak as breathiness.

Fatigue of the voice is the inability to continue to phonate for extended periods without change in vocal quality. The voice may fatigue by becoming hoarse, losing range, changing timbre, breaking into different registers, or by other uncontrolled behaviors. These problems are especially apparent in actors and singers. A well-trained singer should be able to sing for several hours without developing vocal fatigue. Fatigue is often caused by misuse of abdominal and neck musculature or overuse (singing or speaking too loudly or too long). Vocal fatigue also may be a sign of general tiredness, sleep apnea, thyroid abnormalities, myasthenia gravis, or other serious illnesses.

Volume disturbance may present as an inability to speak or sing loudly or softly. Each voice has its own dynamic range. Professional voice users acquire greater loudness through increased vocal efficiency. They learn to speak and sing more softly through years of laborious practice that involves muscle control and development of the ability to use the supraglottic resonators effectively. Most volume problems are secondary to intrinsic limitations of the voice or technical errors in voice production, although hormonal changes, aging and neurological diseases are other causes. Superior laryngeal nerve paresis will impair the ability to speak loudly. This is a frequently unrecognized consequence of viral infection of the laryngeal nerves and may be precipitated by an upper respiratory tract infection.

Even non-singers normally require only about 10 to 30 minutes to warm-up the voice. *Prolonged warm-up time*, especially in the morning, is most often caused by reflux laryngitis, a condition in which stomach acid travels up the esophagus and into the throat, where it causes a chemical burn and symptoms of throat clearing, hoarseness, phlegm, and/or post-nasal drainage, among others.

Tickling or *choking* during speech or singing is often associated with laryngitis or voice abuse. *Pain* while vocalizing can indicate vocal fold lesions, laryngeal joint arthritis, infection, allergies, or acid reflux irritation of the arytenoids, but it is much more commonly caused by voice misuse with excessive muscular activity in the neck.

In evaluating a patient with a voice complaint, the laryngologist will typically ask several questions to help better characterize the nature of the voice complaint and how it is affecting the individual's normal vocal routine.

WHAT IS YOUR VOICE TRAINING AND HOW DO YOU USE YOUR VOICE PROFESSIONALLY?

The amount of voice use and training also affects the voice. Inquiry into vocal habits frequently reveals correctable causes for voice difficulties. Extensive untrained speaking under adverse environmental circumstances is a common example. Such conditions occur, for example, among stock traders who speak over excessive trading room noise, sales people who talk in noisy rooms, restaurant personnel who are required to talk over the background noise of the kitchen and restaurant (and in the presence of significant amounts of cigarette smoke), and people who speak on the telephone in noisy offices.

The problems are aggravated by habits that impair the mechanics of voice production such as sitting with poor posture and bending the neck to hold a telephone against one shoulder. Subconscious efforts to overcome these impediments often produce enough voice abuse to cause vocal fatigue, hoarseness, and even nodules (callous-like growths, usually on both vocal folds). Recognizing and eliminating the causal factors usually result in disappearance of the nodules and an improved voice.

DO YOU SMOKE, USE DRUGS/MEDICATIONS, OR HAVE ANY ENVIRONMENTAL EXPOSURES?

Exposure to environmental irritants is a well-recognized cause of voice dysfunction. Smoke (both primary and second-hand), dehydration, pollution, and allergens may produce hoarseness, frequent throat clearing and vocal fatigue. These problems generally can be eliminated by environmental modification, medication, or simply breathing through the nose rather than the mouth.

Unlike the mouth, the nose warms, humidifies, and filters incoming air, making it of optimal consistency to help lubricate and assist normal vocal fold vibration. Because the mouth is unable to perform these functions, the air that reaches the vocal folds when breathing occurs through the mouth usually is dry, cold, and unfiltered, which can limit lubrication of the vocal folds and make them more susceptible to tearing and hemorrhage from shear forces involved in vocal fold vibration.

The deleterious effects of *tobacco smoke* upon the vocal folds have been known for many years. Smoke from marijuana and other illicit drugs is even more toxic than cigarette smoke and causes more severe injury to the larynx than is typically seen with tobacco smoke. Smoking not only causes chronic irritation but can result in alterations in the vocal fold epithelium (the "skin" cells lining the vocal fold). The epithelial cells change their appearance, becoming more and more different from normal epithelial cells. Eventually, they begin to pile up on each other, rather than lining up in an orderly fashion and can grow rapidly without restraint and invade surrounding tissues. This drastic change is called squamous cell carcinoma, or cancer of the larynx.

The use of various *medications* and *supplements* may affect the voice, too, and it is extremely important for the laryngologist to know all of the prescription and over-the-counter medications that are being taken as well as any herbal remedies, vitamins, supplements or throat sprays that are being used, even if their use is not occurring on a daily basis. Some medications may even permanently ruin a voice, especially androgenic (male) hormones such as those given to women with endometriosis or with post-menopausal sexual dysfunction. Similar problems occur with anabolic steroids (also male hormones) used illicitly by body builders.

More common drugs also can have deleterious vocal effects, but these are usually temporary. Antihistamines, which are used to treat allergies, can cause dryness, increase throat clearing and irritation, and often aggravate hoarseness. Aspirin and other anti-inflammatory pain medications (such as ibuprofen and naproxen) contribute to vocal fold hemorrhages because they decrease the ability of the blood cells to form clots, thus increasing the risk of bleeding. The propellant in inhalers used to treat asthma often produces laryngitis. Many neurological, psychological, and respiratory medications cause tremor that can be heard in the voice. Numerous other medications cause similar problems.

WHAT IS YOUR NORMAL DIET?

Some foods may contribute to voice complaints in people with "normal" vocal folds. Milk products are particularly troublesome to some people. Milk contains casein, which increases and thickens mucosal secretions. Acidic foods, such as tomatoes, lemons, grapefruits, and oranges, aggravate reflux disease, as do caffeine, fried foods, fatty foods, dairy products, and alcohol. Additionally, alcohol can impair one's ability to control the voice, predisposing to vocal injury.

DO YOU HAVE OTHER MEDICAL PROBLEMS?

The history must also assess the status of the respiratory (breathing), cardiovascular (heart and blood vessels), gastrointestinal (stomach and intestines), endocrine (both sex and non-sex hormones), neurological, musculoskeletal, and psychological systems. Disturbances in any of these areas may be responsible for voice complaints. Selected common examples are discussed or illustrated later in this book.

Problems anywhere in the body must be elicited during the medical history. Because voice function relies on complex brain and nervous system interactions, even slight neurological dysfunction may cause voice abnormalities, and voice impairment is sometimes the first symptom of serious neurological diseases (such as myasthenia gravis, multiple sclerosis, Lou Gerhig's disease (also known as amyotrophic lateral sclerosis or ALS), and Parkinson's disease).

Have you Had a Bodily Injury?

A history of a sprained ankle may reveal the true cause of voice dysfunction, especially in a singer, actor, or speaker with great vocal demands. Proper posture is important for optimal function of the abdomen and chest. The imbalance created by standing with the weight over only one foot frequently impairs support enough to cause compensatory vocal strain, leading to hoarseness and voice fatigue. Similar imbalances may occur after other bodily injuries. These include not only injuries that involve support structures, but also problems in the head and neck, especially whiplash injuries.

Naturally, a history of laryngeal trauma or surgery pre-dating voice dysfunction raises concerns about the anatomical integrity of the vocal fold, but a history of interference with the power source through abdominal or thoracic surgery (such as appendectomy, C-section, hysterectomy, and heart surgery) or pregnancy may be just as important in understanding the cause and optimal treatment of vocal problems.

Do you Have Gastrointestinal (GI) Problems?

Gastrointestinal disorders commonly cause voice complaints, and it is important for the treating physician to be aware of a history of such problems, even if that history is remote. The lower esophageal sphincter sits at the entrance to the stomach and is a sling of muscles in the diaphragm that acts as a one-way valve to keep stomach contents in the stomach and to prevent those contents from flowing backward, into the esophagus, when the stomach churns or when abdominal pressure is increased. In reflux laryngitis, stomach acid flows backward from the stomach and through this weak sphincter into the throat, allowing droplets of the irritating gastric acid to come in contact with the vocal folds and even to be aspirated into the lungs in some cases. Reflux may occur with or without a hiatal hernia, which is a medical condition in which the upper part of the stomach lies in the chest, above the lower esophageal sphincter and diaphragm, instead of in its normal position in the abdomen, below the lower esophageal sphincter and diaphragm.

Common symptoms of reflux laryngitis are hoarseness, especially in the morning, prolonged vocal warm-up time, bad breath, sensation of a lump in the throat, post-nasal drainage, mucus or phlegm in the throat, chronic throat tickle, chronic sore throat, cough, a dry mouth, and/or "coated" tongue. Heartburn is frequently absent. Over time, uncontrolled reflux may cause cancer of the esophagus and larynx. So, this condition should be treated aggressively and conscientiously, even in the absence of significant or disabling symptoms.

Do you Have Asthma or Other Problems Breathing?

Respiratory problems are especially problematic to singers, other voice professionals, and wind instrumentalists, but they may cause voice problems in anyone. Appropriate breath support is essential to healthy voice production. The effects of severe respiratory infection are obvious and will not be enumerated. Restrictive lung disease, such as that associated with obesity, may impair support by decreasing lung volume and respiratory efficiency. However, obstructive pulmonary disease, including asthma and chronic obstructive pulmonary disease (COPD) from smoking, are the most common culprits.

Even mild obstructive lung disease can impair breath support enough to cause increased neck and tongue muscle tension and abusive voice use capable of producing vocal fold nodules. This scenario occurs even with unrecognized asthma and may be difficult to diagnose unless suspected, because many such cases of asthma are exercised-induced. Vocal performance is a form of exercise, whether the performance involves singing, giving speeches, sales or other forms of intense voice use. Individuals with exercise-induced asthma will have normal pulmonary function clinically and may even have normal or nearly normal pulmonary function test findings at rest. However, as the voice is used intensively, pulmonary function decreases, effectively impairing support and resulting in compensatory abusive technique. When suspected, this entity can be confirmed through a methacholine challenge test performed by a pulmonary (lung) specialist.

Treatment of the underlying pulmonary disease to restore effective support is essential to resolving the vocal problem. Treating asthma is rendered more difficult in professional voice users because of the need in some patients to avoid inhalers as well as drugs that produce even a mild tremor, which can occur with the most commonly used forms of medications used to treat asthma. The cooperation of a skilled pulmonologist specializing in asthma and sensitive to problems of vocal artists is invaluable.

DO YOU HAVE HORMONAL PROBLEMS?

Hormones are complex, natural chemicals that the body uses to change a variety of bodily functions, including metabolism (how the body uses energy), sexual development, and psychological functioning, to name a few. Endocrine (hormone-related) problems may include thyroid abnormalities, diabetes (elevated blood sugar), other abnormalities in glucose (sugar) metabolism, pituitary (the primary endocrine gland) abnormalities, abnormalities in sex hormone levels, and abnormalities in levels of cortisol (a natural steroid made by the body to help it manage and heal from stress and bodily injury). A dysfunction in any of these hormone systems can have marked vocal effects. These can include the accumulation of fluid in the superficial layer of the lamina propria of the vocal fold, changes in shape of the larynx, changes in the bulk of the muscles in the larynx, changes in the thickness of the vocal folds, and changes in the function of the laryngeal nerves. Any of these changes, which occur from abnormal hormone control, can affect the voice.

Mild *hypothyroidism* (low thyroid hormone levels often associated with goiter) typically causes a muffled voice, slight loss of vocal range, and vocal sluggishness. Similar findings may be seen in *pregnancy*, during use of oral contraceptives (in about 5% of women), for a few days prior to menses, and at the time of ovulation. *Premenstrual* loss of vocal efficiency, endurance and range is also accompanied by a propensity for vocal fold hemorrhage, which may alter the voice permanently. The use of some medications with hormonal activity can also permanently change a voice. This is particularly true of substances that contain androgens (male hormones), which are sometimes used to treat endometriosis.

Hyperthyroidism (elevated thyroid hormone levels) and thyroiditis (inflammation of the thyroid gland) can also be associated with hoarseness, usually due to inflammation surrounding the laryngeal nerves, which may manifest as breathiness, vocal instability, voice breaks, vocal fatigue, difficulty producing a loud volume, and difficulty with vocal projection. Similarly, *diabetes* may cause a peripheral neuropathy (abnormal nerve function) that may involve the laryngeal nerves and contribute to vocal fold paresis. Syndromes associated with abnormal *cortisol* levels may cause the abnormal accumulation of fluid in the vocal folds and loss of normal vocal fold vibration, increased raspiness, voice breaks, and difficulty controlling the voice.

Any prior history of thyroid problems, irregular menstrual periods, heavy menstrual periods, missed menstrual periods, spotting, ovarian cysts or other ovarian abnormalities, difficulties with fertility, history of diabetes, history of low blood sugar (hypoglycemia), history of abnormal cortisol production (Cushing's syndrome or Addison's disease), abnormal or inappropriate milk production from the breasts, breast cancer, testosterone problems, difficulties with achieving or maintaining erection, testicular cancer, prostate problems, or other hormone-related problems should be discussed with the laryngologist because of this complex interaction between hormones and the voice.

The Examination

Following the medical history, the physician will perform a physical examination, which includes examination of the entire ear, nose, throat, head, and neck region. Included in this evaluation should be an assessment of hearing function. This should include at least examination with a tuning fork and, if indicated, a formal hearing test (audiogram). After the head and neck are examined, a detailed assessment of the larynx is usually performed.

Evaluation of the larynx usually involves evaluation of the movement of the vocal folds during speech, singing, and other tasks and evaluation of the vibratory function of the folds. Vocal fold movement is usually best assessed with a flexible, fiberoptic laryngoscope with continuous light, and assessment of vocal fold vibration is usually assessed with stroboscopic light, using either a flexible laryngoscope, a rigid laryngoscope, or both.

FLEXIBLE LARYNGOSCOPIC EXAMINATION

A flexible laryngoscope is a thin, lighted telescope (endoscope) that is placed through the nose and into the throat. It usually does not cause pain, although it may cause a slight discomfort in the nose. The patient is seated and awake during the examination. The flexible laryngoscope allows the physician to see the larynx in its natural position. In this way, the physician can assess changes in laryngeal muscle tension while the patient is talking or singing.

There are certain vocal maneuvers that the otolaryngologist or laryngologist will ask the patient to perform during the flexible laryngoscopic examination.

These include various tasks of talking, singing, and whistling. While the patient is performing these maneuvers, the doctor is evaluating the motion and mobility of the vocal folds.

The patient will be asked to perform several tasks that require stretching and lengthening of the vocal folds. These tasks may include counting at several different pitches and/or sliding from a low pitch to a high pitch while saying the sound /i/. If there is a primary problem in the superior laryngeal nerve, this will be evidenced by an inability to lengthen the vocal fold with high-pitched phonation. If the weakness is severe, there can be a tilt of the larynx toward the side of the weakened superior laryngeal nerve and/or cricothyroid muscle. The larynx tilts toward the side of the weakness on lengthening because the cricothyroid muscle on the normal side pulls the thyroid cartilage anteriorly (forward) and down toward the cricoid cartilage; the paretic cricothyroid muscle is weak and pulls the thyroid cartilage to a lesser degree, resulting in tilting of the larynx toward the side of the weak superior laryngeal nerve and cricothyroid muscle.

If there are problems with both superior laryngeal nerves, there will be limitations in the ability to produce a high pitch and in the ability to stretch the vocal folds on both sides.[3] This diagnosis may be somewhat difficult, especially if both nerves are injured to the same degree. Both vocal folds will have limitations in their abilities to stretch, making the ability to see subtle abnormalities difficult for the examiner.

Occasionally, with superior laryngeal nerve paresis, an abnormality is seen in the ability of the vocal fold on the affected side to close. Sluggish closure of the vocal fold is best seen when the patient tries to engage in vocal maneuvers that involve a rapid movement of the vocal folds. These vocal maneuvers involve performing such repetitive tasks as saying /i/-/hi/, alternating a quick sniff with saying /i/, saying /pa/-/ta/-/ka/. Because the ability to do these maneuvers involves the rapid movement of the vocal folds, subtle differences in vocal fold motion are easily revealed.

If the recurrent laryngeal nerve is injured, there may be abnormalities in closing and opening of the vocal folds. The posterior cricoarytenoid muscle opens the vocal folds. The thyroarytenoid, interarytenoid, lateral cricoarytenoid, and, to a lesser degree, the cricothyroid muscles close the vocal folds. Abnormalities in the ability to close the vocal folds are evaluated by the same maneuvers as stated above.

Differentiating problems with the superior laryngeal nerve versus the recurrent laryngeal nerve when impaired or sluggish closure is seen can be difficult. In general, if the problem is with the superior laryngeal nerve, one should also see problems with tensing and stretching the vocal folds. If the problem is with the recurrent laryngeal nerve, problems with closure alone or in combination with difficulties in opening the vocal folds, but not tensing or stretching the vocal folds, should be seen.

Abnormalities in opening the vocal folds are frequently evaluated by having the patient sniff and whistle. Both of these maneuvers require that the vocal folds open briskly. If the recurrent laryngeal nerve is injured at its insertion into the posterior cricoarytenoid muscle, the vocal fold will have problems with opening only. If the injury to the nerve occurs at the level of the thyroarytenoid or lateral cricoarytenoid muscles, there will be isolated abnormalities in closing the vocal folds. If there is a

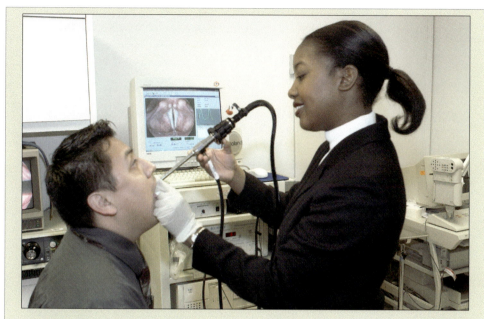

FIGURE 6–1. A rigid strobovideolaryngoscopic examination.

problem with the nerve at any point before it enters the larynx, there will be abnormalities in both opening and closing the vocal folds.

When the muscles are completely paralyzed or near totally paralyzed, the vocal folds do not move on the side that is affected; however, a Jostle's sign is seen. A Jostle's sign is a movement of the arytenoid cartilage on the affected side during vocalization. The passive movement of the arytenoid on the affected side occurs as a result of contact with the other arytenoid, which presses against it during vocal fold closure.

If the abnormality is in the movement of the cricoarytenoid joint and not in the vocal fold muscles or nerves, the vocal fold will have sluggish or absent movement, but there will be evidence of some muscular effort (as long as there is not associated muscle or nerve injury). This muscular effort is typically seen as a tensing of the thyroarytenoid muscle during vocal maneuvers without a concomitant change in the position of the vocal fold.

RIGID STROBOVIDEOLARYNGOSCOPY

Rigid strobovideolaryngoscopy allows a more magnified and optically superior view of the vibratory function and structure of the vocal fold. Strobovideolaryngoscopy involves the use of synchronized flashing lights through an endoscope to evaluate the function of the mucosal wave of the vocal fold. This procedure is performed with a rigid laryngoscope placed through the mouth with the tongue held forward (Figure 6-1). The patient is awake and seated in a forward position during the examination. The chin is held slightly upright in a "sniffing" position, which helps to pull the base of the tongue forward so that the larynx can be viewed more easily. Occasionally, a sensation of gagging is experienced during the examination; otherwise, the examination does not cause much discomfort. This magnified view of the vocal folds can give the physician information regarding structural lesions on the vocal folds that may contribute to the vocal complaint or that have arisen as a result of the paresis.

Once a movement disorder of the larynx is identified, laryngeal electromyography (LEMG) is ordered to help examine more accurately the integrity of the neuromotor (nerve and muscle) system. Laboratory studies, biopsies, and imaging studies may help guide the diagnosis and management of movement disorders as well.

Laryngeal Electromyography (LEMG)

Laryngeal electromyography (LEMG) is a procedure that evaluates the integrity of the muscular and nervous systems of the larynx. This test is performed on patients who have evidence of a movement disorder of the vocal folds. The purpose of the LEMG is to help the physician diagnose and differentiate the causes of these movement disorders.

There are several different types of problems that can result in abnormal motions of the vocal folds. These can be classified as disorders in movements of the joints that connect the cartilages of the larynx, primary problems within the muscles themselves, or problems in the nerves that supply the muscles of the larynx. Understanding the exact mechanism of the problem is important in helping the physician understand how to treat the patient's voice problems best and in helping speech-language pathologists and singing voice therapists select the best exercises to help rehabilitate the voice.

When a person makes a decision to vocalize, the brain initiates the phonation by sending an electrical signal to the brainstem, which then transfers the impulse through the recurrent and superior laryngeal nerves. As the electrical impulse reaches the end of the nerve, it signals the release of a substance called a neurotransmitter from the tip of the nerve. In the larynx, the predominant neurotransmitter is a chemical called acetylcholine. As this neurotransmitter is released from the end of the nerve, it binds to its receptor on the muscle, causing chemicals to be released inside the muscle that signal the muscle to contract. The contraction of the muscle then produces the movements of the vocal folds, resulting in voice production as air is forced from the lungs through the closing vocal folds.

LEMG takes advantage of the fact that the nerve has an electrical signal that is transferred to a chemical signal at the muscle receptor (called the neuromuscular junction). During LEMG, electrodes are placed in the muscles of the larynx. These electrodes sense the electrical impulses within the muscle and transpose them to a visual and auditory signal that can be interpreted by the physician or an electrophysiologist (a professional who is trained in the interpretation of electrical signals from the body) who is performing the study. The information gained from the LEMG helps in the differentiation and diagnosis of disorders in nerve, muscle, and joint function.

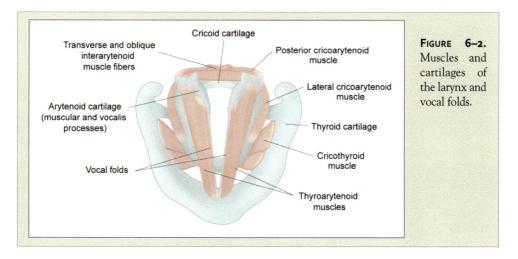

FIGURE 6-2. Muscles and cartilages of the larynx and vocal folds.

HOW IS LEMG DONE?

LEMG is often performed as a diagnostic procedure, but it also can be performed therapeutically to help guide the placement of botulinum toxin. Botulinum toxin, whose tradename is Botox™, is a toxin produced by the bacteria that cause botulism. Medicinally, it is used to weaken hyperactive muscles. The procedure of LEMG is the same regardless of whether is it for diagnostic purposes or for guidance for injection of botulinum toxin.

Because neurologists, physiatrists, and electrophysiologists perform electromyography (EMG) on other parts of the body on a daily basis, and because their professional training equips them with expertise to interpret complex signals, many otolaryngologists and laryngologists prefer to obtain their opinions in the interpretation of diagnostic LEMGs. Because the use of LEMG for botulinum toxin injections into laryngeal muscles requires a level of expertise in laryngeal anatomy, physiology, and LEMG interpretation that most otolaryngologists and laryngologists receive in their professional training, LEMG for botulinum toxin injections is often performed solely by these physicians.

To perform LEMG, the patient is usually asked to lie down with the chin held upwards and the head tilted back. This position helps to bring the larynx closer to the skin, making it easier to insert the electrodes into the laryngeal muscles. The neck is cleaned with alcohol to prevent the introduction of any infectious materials on the skin into the larynx. The insertion of the needle electrodes through the skin feels like a pinprick; the insertion into the muscles of the larynx produces a small, sharp stabbing sensation, similar to the sensation experienced while getting a tetanus shot. Local anesthetic can be given to prevent the pinprick sensation on the skin, but it cannot be given for the sensations experienced during insertion of the electrodes into the muscles. The presence of the anesthetic will alter the electrical signals of the nerves and muscles, confounding the results.

There are four pairs of muscle groups in the larynx: the thyroarytenoid, the lateral cricoarytenoid, the posterior cricoarytenoid, and the cricothyroid muscles (Figure 6-2). The interarytenoid muscle sits in the midline of the back of the larynx and is not paired. Usually, the thyroarytenoid, the posterior cricoarytenoid, and the cricothyroid muscles are tested on each side. Testing of these three groups of muscles usually gives sufficient information about the integrity of the superior and recurrent laryngeal nerves and the muscles that they innervate. When equivocal results are obtained or when special information is needed, the lateral cricoarytenoid and the interarytenoid muscles may be tested as well.

To test the muscles, the physician positions the needle in the direction of the muscle of interest. When the physician feels as though the needle is positioned correctly, the patient is asked to perform laryngeal maneuvers (phonating, sniffing, breathing, or swallowing) that require contraction of the muscle of interest and relative relaxation of other muscles of the larynx. When the muscle contracts, the electrical signal seen on the monitor and the auditory signal heard through the speaker will be increased with the appropriate maneuver. If botulinum toxin is to be injected, it is injected through the EMG needle at this time.

If there is evidence of weakness, repetitive stimulation studies and possible Tensilon™ testing may be performed. Repetitive stimulation involves stimulating a nerve with electrical shocks and recording the neuromuscular response by EMG. The nerve stimulated is often the spinal accessory nerve, which moves the trapezius muscle, one of the large muscles of the shoulder. This nerve is chosen because it lies just beneath the skin in the neck and is easy to locate for stimulation. Many people describe the sensation experienced during repetitive stimulation studies as being similar to the sensation of an electrical shock going from the shoulder through the arm. Repetitive stimulation gives information regarding the integrity of the neuromuscular junctions in general.

If this test is abnormal or if other abnormalities are seen on the LEMG, Tensilon™ testing may be performed. A drug named edrophonium, whose tradename is Tensilon™, is injected into a vein, and the LEMG is repeated. Tensilon™ testing helps to determine whether the site of the problem is in the nerve-muscle interface (the neuromuscular junction). When it is injected into the vein, a needle prick is felt; otherwise there are no other abnormal sensations. The sensations experienced during the LEMG for Tensilon™ testing are similar to the sensations experienced during the first LEMG.

How Are the LEMG Data Used?

At the completion of the LEMG, the physician has valuable information that will help to guide his or her diagnosis of the laryngeal mobility problems. Each of the factors investigated with the LEMG helps to give the physician an indication of the duration of the problem, its cause, and the likelihood that the problem will worsen, improve, or remain stable. Sometimes, serial LEMGs are needed to follow changes in nerve recovery or decline over time, which may help to give a better prediction of nerve function in the future.

In patients with paresis and/or paralysis, the results of the LEMG may also help to guide subsequent therapy. If paresis is found, the patient can undergo voice therapy that is specifically aimed at increasing the strength of the weak muscle. In patients with abnormalities in vocal fold mobility who may benefit from surgical procedures to enhance their vocal function, the LEMG can help to determine the nature and timing of the surgical procedure. If there is evidence of ongoing nerve damage, surgery may be delayed until the damage is complete. Similarly, if there is evidence of recovery, surgery may be delayed until maximal recovery has been achieved.

Vocal Function Testing

Part of the diagnosis of voice disorders involves measuring various aerodynamic, subjective, and physical characteristics of the voice. Vocal function testing is usually performed by the voice scientist in the voice lab but may also involve questionnaires that the patient completes individually. The purpose of vocal function testing is to evaluate how the patient is affected by his or her voice problem in daily activities (subjective measures) and to quantify the voice in a manner that will allow comparison over time (objective measures) and assessment of how the voice responds to treatment.

PATIENT REPORT INDICES

Patient report indices allow the laryngologist to determine the effects of voice disorders on the patient's normal activities of daily living and, thus, measure the degree of handicap the voice disorder poses to the patient. Often, patients are asked to complete these questionnaires prior to seeing the physician. The most popular of these include the Voice Handicap Index, the Voice Related Quality of Life, the Voice Outcome Survey, and the Glottal Closure Index, among others. Each of these measures asks the patient questions about the emotional, physical, and functional impacts of his or her voice disorder, the results of which help to guide the treatment plan.

OBJECTIVE VOICE MEASURES

Objective measures of vocal function are usually performed in the voice laboratory by the voice scientist. These measures seek to quantify perceptual characteristics of the voice, thus, allowing evaluation of changes in "normality" of the voice by comparing values obtained from the patient with known "normal" values. These can be valuable in correlating perceptual observations of vocal function with objective assessment and can help to assess the potential for rehabilitation as well as the effect of treatment on vocal function.

The two main categories of objective voice measures are aerodynamic measures and measures of acoustic analysis.

Aerodynamic Measures

Aerodynamic measures of vocal function evaluate the mechanics of airflow in voice production. They include spirometry, glottal airflow rate, subglottal air pressure, maximum phonation time, and calculation of the s/z ratio.

Spirometry

Spirometry, or pulmonary function testing as it is also commonly known, measures lung function and gives an indication of the degree of airway opening or narrowing. These measures are important in assessing pulmonary (lung) and tracheal (windpipe) contributions to disordered voice production. Limitations in pulmonary function (such as occur with asthma and emphysema) can restrict the ability to build enough pressure to cause efficient vocal fold vibration and a normal voice.

With spirometry, usually the patient is asked to inhale and exhale into a tube that is connected to a machine that measures the volume of air that is exchanged. Various tasks, designed to measure lung capacity and lung volumes during various degrees of inhalation and exhalation are measured with the spirometry.

Glottal Airflow Rate

Measures of glottal airflow rate allow the voice scientist to assess the degree of air movement across the vocal folds during phonation and, thus, reflect the integrity of the vocal tract. The mean airflow rate during sustained phonation of a vowel is the best indicator of the functional efficiency of the vocal folds. These measurements are obtained using a facemask that collects oral airflow and a flow transducer attached to the facemask that measures airflow. The facemask is placed over the mouth and nose to create a seal, and the patient is asked to perform various vocal tasks, which are measured and recorded by the flow transducer and a computer interface.

Subglottal Air Pressure

Subglottal air pressure is the energy required in the subglottis (the area below the vocal folds) to force open the vocal folds in sound production. This pressure correlates with the sound pressure level (volume) produced and should increase with greater vocal volume and decrease with the production of softer sounds. An elevated subglottal pressure for a given volume implies vocal fold or supraglottic hyperfunction or constriction. Inadequate or unstable pressure regulation may result in a soft voice and may signal pulmonary, chest wall, or vocal fold disorders. Subglottal air pressure is also measured with a facemask and transducer.

Maximum Phonation Time

The maximum phonation time is the longest length of time that a patient can sustain phonation of a vowel. The patient is asked to take a deep breath, voice a vowel, usually /a/, and hold that vowel sound for as long as possible. The voice scientist measures the length of time between the onset and end of phonation. Usually, the patient is given three tries, and the longest of the three tries is the maximum phonation time. It is a very crude measure of airflow through the vocal folds. The basic assumption of the measure is that the more efficient the vocal fold mechanism, the longer the maximum phonation time will be. The maximum phonation time is a good therapeutic tool for patients, allowing them to track progress at home.

s/z RATIO

The s/z ratio compares the maximal amount of time a patient can produce the sound /s/ versus the maximal amount of time he or she can produce the sound /z/. The theory behind the ratio is that production of the sound /s/ depends primarily on lung function, breath control, and breath support, whereas production of the sound /z/ depends on these as well as appropriate vocal fold vibratory efficiency. Thus, a normal individual should be able to produce the /s/ and the /z/ for similar lengths of time, giving a normal s/z ratio at about one. In patients with a gap between their vocal folds, the duration of the /z/ is expected to be less than that of the /s/, giving a larger ratio. The s/z ratio is best used to track individual changes in vocal production through time

Acoustic Analysis

Acoustic analysis is the analysis of the energy characteristics of the voice that relate to pitch, loudness, and vocal quality. The goal of acoustic analysis is to measure in a meaningful way perceptual characteristics of the voice.

FREQUENCY RANGE

Determination of the fundamental frequency of phonation gives an indication of the primary rate of vibration of the vocal folds during normal conversational speech. The frequency range is determined by having the patient phonate from the middle of their range up to his or her highest attainable note and again down to the lowest attainable note. The patient phonates into a microphone, and a voice analysis software program calculates the frequency of phonation. The frequency range gives an indication of pliability of the vocal folds as well as of vocal fold muscle functions. Changes in frequency range can be used to assess the effectiveness of therapy, particularly in patients with vocal fold stiffness, scarring, or paresis.

SOUND PRESSURE LEVEL

Sound pressure level measurements usually are obtained from samples of speech and are used as indicators of habitual loudness. The patient is asked to speak into a microphone. The speech is recorded and analyzed by a computer software program that indicates the mean sound pressure level (loudness) of the speech sample as well as the loudness of different areas of speech. The sound pressure level measurements often serve as indicators of the patient's ability to monitor the volume of the speaking voice and can be helpful as biofeedback tools in voice therapy.

SPECTRAL ANALYSIS

Spectral analysis involves the measurement of the energy characteristics of the voice throughout the frequency spectrum and calculation of the degree of harmonic structure of the voice. Every sound is composed of many sound waves. Spectral analysis evaluates the energy patterns in the voice during speech and evaluates the degree of harmony (clarity) and perturbation (noise). With spectral analysis, the patient is asked to phonate various vocal tasks into a microphone. The voice sample is recorded by a computer software program, which then calculates the spectral (energy and frequency) characteristics of the voice signal.

Vocal function tests are useful adjuncts to the evaluation and treatment of voice disorders. They allow for objective measurement of the voice and vocal function and the ability to follow changes in the voice through time. Vocal function testing is best used as a battery of cognitive, behavioral, physical, acoustic, and aerodynamic evaluation to provide a global view of vocal function.

Voice Evaluation and Voice Therapy

Once the laryngologist has completed the evaluation and made a medical diagnosis, he or she often recommends evaluation by a voice therapist. The purpose of the voice therapy evaluation is to examine behavioral habits that have developed in response to the voice problem and that may have contributed to the development of the voice problem. The voice therapist will also evaluate the breath support mechanism, intonation, use of laryngeal and extralaryngeal muscles, vocal projection, resonance patterns, and the mechanism of volume and pitch control during singing and speaking.

Voice abuse through technical dysfunction is an extremely common source of hoarseness, vocal weakness, pain, and other complaints. In some cases, voice abuse can even create structural problems, such as vocal nodules, cysts, and polyps. Now that the components of voice function are better understood, techniques have been developed to rehabilitate and train the voice in speech and singing. Such voice therapy improves breathing and abdominal support, decreases excess muscle activity in the larynx and neck, optimizes the mechanics of glottal airflow, and maximizes the contributions of the resonance cavities. It also teaches vocal hygiene, including techniques to eliminate voice strain and abuse, maintain hydration and mucosal function, mitigate the effects of smoke and other environmental irritants, and optimize vocal and general health.

Progress is monitored not only by listening to the patient and observing the disappearance of laryngeal pathology when it is present, but also by quantitative measurement in the clinical voice laboratory. However, in some cases there are structural problems in the larynx that are correctable only with surgery.

Summary

The visit with the laryngologist should entail a thorough evaluation of the voice and possible contributors to the voice problem. This should include a thorough history and physical examination, laryngoscopic examination, videostroboscopy, vocal function testing, speech therapy evaluation, and, when appropriate, singing voice therapy evaluation, laryngeal electromyography, blood testing, and radiographic imaging. It is equally important for the patient to be thorough in relaying an accurate history of the voice problem as well as other, seemingly nonrelated medical problems to the physician as it is for the physician to perform a thorough evaluation. At the conclusion of the evaluation, a good, basic understanding of all of the contributing factors underlying the voice problem should be obtained and steps toward treatment should be instituted.

7 What Are the Possible Causes of My Voice Problem?

Difficulties with the voice can arise from both medical and functional disorders. These can include vocal fold masses, neurologic abnormalities that affect the larynx, muscular abnormalities involving the laryngeal muscles, infection, hormonal imbalances, metabolic imbalances (such as diabetes), trauma, and medical conditions that affect other bodily systems and either directly or indirectly affect the voice.

What is Hoarseness?

Most people with voice problems complain of "hoarseness" or "laryngitis." A more accurate description of the problem is often helpful in identifying the cause.

Hoarseness is a coarse, scratchy sound caused most commonly by abnormalities on the vibratory margin of the vocal fold. These may include swelling, roughness from inflammation, growths, scarring, or anything that interferes with symmetric, rhythmic vocal fold vibration. Such abnormalities produce turbulence, which we perceive as hoarseness.

Breathiness is caused by lesions (abnormalities) that keep the vocal folds from closing completely, including paralysis/paresis (immobile or weak vocal folds), muscle weakness, stiffness of the cricoarytenoid joint from injury or arthritis, vocal fold masses, or atrophy (loss of bulk or thickness) of the vocal fold tissues. These abnormalities permit air to escape when the vocal folds are supposed to be tightly closed. We hear this air leak as breathiness.

Fatigue of the voice is the inability to continue to phonate for extended periods without a change in vocal quality. The voice may fatigue by becoming hoarse, los-

---

Modified in part from Sataloff RT. *Professional Voice: The Science and Art of Clinical Care*, 3rd edition. San Diego, California: Plural Publishing, Inc.; 2005 (with permission).

ing range, losing volume, changing timbre, breaking into different registers, or by other uncontrolled behavior. These problems are especially apparent in actors and singers. A well-trained singer should be able to sing for several hours without developing vocal fatigue. Fatigue is often caused by misuse of abdominal and neck musculature or overuse (singing or speaking too loudly, too long). Vocal fatigue may be a sign of general tiredness or of serious illnesses such as myasthenia gravis.

Volume disturbance (loudness) may present as an inability to speak or sing loudly or an inability to phonate softly. Each voice has its own dynamic range. Professional voice users acquire greater loudness through increased vocal efficiency. They learn to speak and sing more softly through years of laborious practice that involves muscle control and the development of the ability to use the supraglottic resonators effectively. Most volume problems are secondary to intrinsic limitations of the voice or technical errors in voice production, although hormonal changes, aging, and neurological disease are other causes. Superior laryngeal nerve paresis or paralysis will impair the ability to speak loudly. This is a frequently unrecognized consequence of viral infections, including those caused by the herpes virus (such as "cold sores") or the influenza virus (such as the flu), and may be precipitated by an upper respiratory tract infection.

Even nonsingers normally require only about 10 to 30 minutes to warm-up the voice. *Prolonged warm-up* time, especially in the morning, is most often caused by reflux laryngitis, a condition in which stomach acid travels backward from the stomach and up the esophagus to the larynx and nasopharynx, where it "burns" the throat. *Tickling* or *choking* during speech or singing is often associated with reflux laryngitis.

A *sudden change* in the voice while speaking or singing is often a symptom of a disorder affecting the vocal fold's leading edge(such as a vocal fold hemorrhage or tear). This symptom requires that voice use be avoided until vocal fold examination has been accomplished.

Pain while vocalizing can indicate vocal fold lesions, laryngeal joint arthritis, infection, or gastric (stomach) acid reflux irritation of the arytenoids; but it is much more commonly caused by voice abuse with excessive muscular activity in the neck, rather than acute pathology on the leading edge of a vocal fold, and it does not usually require immediate cessation of phonation pending medical examination.

Does Age Affect the Voice?

Age affects the voice significantly, especially during childhood and in advanced age. Children's voices are particularly fragile. Voice abuse during childhood may lead to problems that persist throughout a lifetime. It is extremely important for children to learn good vocal habits and for them to avoid voice abuse. This is especially true among children who choose to participate in vocally taxing activities such as singing, acting and cheerleading. Many promising careers and vocal avocations have been ruined by enthusiastic but untrained voice use. For children with vocal interests, age-appropriate training should be started early. Any child with unexplained or prolonged hoarseness should undergo prompt, expert medical evaluation performed by a laryngologist (ear, nose and throat doctor) specializing in voice care.

In older patients, vocal unsteadiness, loss of range, and voice fatigue may be associated with typical changes of normal aging, such as vocal fold atrophy (wasting). In routine speech, such vocal changes allow a person to be identified as "old" even over the telephone. Among singers, they are typically associated with flat pitch and a "wobble" often heard in older amateur choir singers. However, recent evidence has shown that many of these voice changes are not caused by irreversible aging changes. Rather, they may be consequences of poor laryngeal, respiratory, and abdominal muscle conditioning (that also changes with age) undermining the power source of the voice. The medical history usually reveals minimal aerobic exercise and shortness of breath on climbing stairs or walking long distances. With appropriate conditioning of the body and voice, many of the characteristics associated with vocal aging can be eliminated, and a youthful sound can be restored.

What Are the Effects of Voice Use and Training?

The amount of voice use and training also affects voices. Inquiry into vocal habits frequently reveals correctable causes for voice difficulties. Extensive untrained speaking under adverse environmental circumstances is a common example. Such conditions occur, for example, among stock traders, sales people, restaurant personnel, and people who speak over the telephone in noisy offices. The problems are aggravated by habits that impair the mechanics of voice production, such as sitting with poor posture and bending the neck to hold a telephone against one shoulder. Subconscious efforts to overcome these impediments often produce enough voice abuse to cause vocal fatigue, hoarseness, and even nodules (callous-like growths on the vocal folds). Recognizing and eliminating the causal factors usually results in disappearance of the nodules and improved voice.

Professional singers, actors, announcers, politicians, and other voice professionals put "Olympic" demands on their voices. Interest in the diagnosis and treatment of special problems of professional voice users is responsible for the evolution of voice care as a subspecialty of otolaryngology. These patients are often managed best by subspecialists familiar with the latest concepts in professional voice care.

How About Smoke and Other Things in the Air?

Exposure to *environmental irritants* is a well-recognized cause of voice dysfunction. Smoke, dehydration, pollution, and allergens may produce hoarseness, frequent throat clearing, and voice fatigue. These problems can generally be eliminated by environmental modification, medication, or simply breathing through the nose rather than the mouth (since the nose warms, humidifies, and filters incoming air).

Stage fogs and pyrotechnic effects also can cause irritation that affects the voice and lungs.

The deleterious effects of *tobacco smoke* upon the vocal folds have been known for many years. Smoking not only causes chronic irritation, but moreover it can result in histologic (microscopic) alterations in the vocal fold epithelium (the lining tissue). The epithelial cells change their appearance, becoming more and more different from normal epithelial cells. Eventually, they begin to pile up on each other, rather than lining up in an orderly fashion. Eventually, they escape normal control mechanisms in the body and begin to grow rapidly, without restraint, and invade surrounding tissues. This drastic change is called squamous cell carcinoma, or cancer of the larynx.

Can Foods or Drugs Affect the Voice?

The use of various foods and drugs may affect the voice, too. Some medications may even permanently ruin a voice, especially androgenic (male) hormones such as those given to women with endometriosis or with post-menopausal sexual dysfunction. Similar problems occur with anabolic steroids (also male hormones) used illicitly by body builders and athletes to enhance muscle performance.

More common drugs also have deleterious vocal effects, usually temporary. *Antihistamines* cause dryness, increased throat clearing and irritation, and often aggravate hoarseness. *Aspirin*, ibuprofen, naproxen, and other anti-inflammatory pain killers (NSAIDs) contribute to vocal fold hemorrhages by the same anti-clotting effect that makes them a good drug for patients with heart disease, high cholesterol, and vascular (blood vessel) disease. The propellant in inhalers used to treat *asthma* often produces laryngitis, and many steroid asthma medications can cause chronic thrush infections on the vocal folds as well as lead to atrophy (wasting) of the vocal folds. Many neurological, psychological, and respiratory medications cause tremor that can be heard in the voice. Numerous other medications cause similar problems.

Some foods may also be responsible for voice complaints in people with "normal" vocal folds. Milk products are particularly troublesome to some people because the casein they contain increases and thickens mucosal secretions, causing a sensation of mucous and phlegm in the throat.

What General Health and Medical Conditions Can Affect the Voice?

Problems anywhere in the body can cause voice dysfunction. For example, because voice function relies on complex brain and other nervous system interactions, even slight neurological dysfunction may cause voice abnormalities; and voice impairment is sometimes the first symptom of serious neurological diseases such as stroke, myasthenia gravis, multiple sclerosis, ALS (Lou Gherig's disease), and Parkinson's disease.

A history of a sprained ankle may reveal the true cause of voice dysfunction, especially in a singer, actor, or speaker with great vocal demands. Proper posture is important to optimal function of the abdomen and chest. The imbalance created by standing with the weight over only one foot frequently impairs support enough to cause compensatory vocal strain, leading to hoarseness and voice fatigue. Similar imbalances may occur after other bodily injuries. These include not only injuries that involve support structures, but also problems in the head and neck, especially whiplash injuries.

Naturally, a history of laryngeal trauma or surgery predating voice dysfunction raises concerns about the anatomical integrity of the vocal fold, but a history of interference with the power source through neck, abdominal, or chest surgery may be just as important in understanding the cause and optimal treatment of vocal problems.

CAN HEARING LOSS AFFECT THE VOICE?

Singers and actors typically modulate their voices by listening to them. Auditory feedback is important, as is the ability to hear fellow performers. Hearing loss is a common source of voice problems, and it is often overlooked. Hearing loss can cause vocal strain, particularly if a person has sensorineural hearing loss (involving the nerve or inner ear) and is unaware of it. This condition may lead people to speak or sing more loudly than they realize.

Voice professionals also should avoid very loud noise that can damage hearing and should have their hearing tested periodically. Chronic exposure to loud noise is a common cause of hearing loss, including the use of earbuds with MP3 player, performing in front of loud bands, and improperly balanced feedback monitors. Singers who perform with loud bands should use a custom-fitted noise-reducing earplugs with a built-in feedback monitor. These can be fitted and made by an audiologist who specializes in the needs of performing artists.

DO ALLERGY AND POST-NASAL DRIP BOTHER THE VOICE?

Allergies and post-nasal drip alter the viscosity (thickness) of mucous secretions, the degree of opening of the nasal passages, and have other effects that impair voice use. Many of the medicines commonly used to treat allergies (such as antihistamines) have undesirable effects on the voice. When allergies are severe enough to cause persistent throat clearing, hoarseness, and other voice complaints despite the use of non-antihistamine allergy medications, a comprehensive allergy evaluation and treatment is advisable.

"Post-nasal drip," the sensation of excessive secretions, may or may not be caused by allergy or sinus disease. Contrary to popular opinion, post-nasal drainage usually is caused by secretions which are too thick, rather than too thin or abundant, and can be caused by allergies, reflux, sinusitis, deviated septum, or rhinitis (chronic nasal inflammation). If post-nasal drip is not caused by allergy, it is usually managed best through hydration and agents designed to thin the secretions.

Reflux laryngitis can cause symptoms very similar to post-nasal drip, and it should always be considered in people who have the sensation of throat secretions, a lump in the throat, and excessive throat clearing.

WHAT IS THE EFFECT OF UPPER RESPIRATORY TRACT INFECTIONS (WITHOUT LARYNGITIS)?

Although mucosal irritation from an upper respiratory tract infection usually is diffuse, patients sometimes have marked nasal obstruction with little or no sore throat and a "normal" voice. If the laryngeal examination shows no abnormality, a person with a "head cold" should be permitted to speak or sing, advised not to try to duplicate his or her usual sound, but rather to accept the insurmountable alteration caused by the change from the infection in the supraglottic vocal tract and to temporarily alter the repertoire performed, until the cold resolves. This is especially important in singers. The decision as to whether performing under these circumstances is advisable professionally rests with the singer. Throat clearing should be avoided, as this is traumatic to the vocal folds. If a cough is present, medications should be used to suppress it.

HOW ABOUT LARYNGITIS?

Infectious laryngitis may be caused by bacteria or viruses. Subglottic involvement frequently indicates a more severe infection, which may be difficult to control in a short period of time. Indiscriminate use of antibiotics must be prevented. However, when the physician is in doubt as to the cause and when a major voice commitment is imminent, vigorous antibiotic treatment is warranted. Corticosteroids (steroids) may also be helpful in selected cases; these are different from anabolic steroids that have gained notoriety through abuse by athletes.

Mild to moderate edema (swelling) and erythema (redness) of the vocal folds may result from infection or from noninfectious causes. In the absence of vocal fold tearing or hemorrhage, mild to moderate edema and erythema are not absolute contraindications to voice use. Noninfectious laryngitis commonly is associated with excessive voice use in pre-performance rehearsals. It also may be caused by other forms of voice abuse and by mucosal irritation produced by allergy, stage smoke, cigarette smoke, and other causes. Laryngitis sicca (dry throat) is associated with dehydration, dry atmosphere, mouth breathing, and antihistamine therapy. It may also be a symptom of diabetes and other medical problems. Deficiency of lubrication causes irritation and coughing and results in mild inflammation.

If no pressing professional need for voice use exists, inflammatory conditions of the larynx are best treated with relative voice rest in addition to other modalities. However, in some instances speaking or singing may be permitted. The more professional voice training a person has, the safer it will be to use the voice under adverse circumstances. The patient should be instructed to avoid all forms of irritation and to rest the voice at all times except during warm-up and performance. Corticosteroids and other medications discussed later may be helpful. If mucosal secretions are excessive, low-dose antihistamine therapy may be beneficial, but it must be prescribed with caution and should generally be avoided. Copious, thin

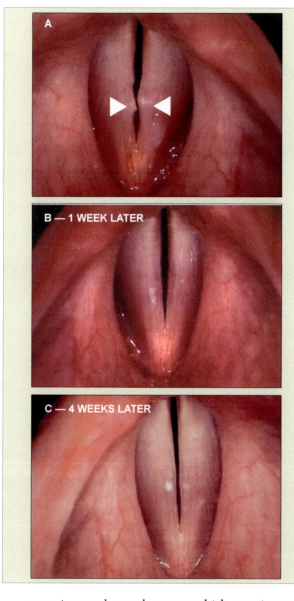

Figure 7–1. A, Bilateral vocal fold tears (*arrows*) and diffuse inflammation in an opera singer who developed hoarseness and the tear from coughing during an upper respiratory tract infection; **B,** with resolution after 1 week of voice rest; **C,** after 4 weeks of voice rest, both the tear and the inflammation have resolved.

secretions are better than scant, thick secretions or excessive dryness. Individuals with laryngitis must be kept well hydrated to maintain the desired character of vocal fold lubrication.

Severe inflammation and swelling, hemorrhage in the vocal folds, and mucosal disruption (a tear) may occur with laryngitis and are absolute contraindications to voice use (Figure 7-1). When these are observed, the treatment includes strict voice rest in addition to correction of any underlying disease. Vocal fold hemorrhage is most common in premenstrual women who are using aspirin products or non-steroidal anti-inflammatory medications such as ibuprofen (trade names Motrin™ and Advil™) or naproxen (trade names Naprosyn™ and Aleve™), but can occur in anyone who overexerts his or her voice. Severe hemorrhage and mucosal scarring may result in permanent hoarseness. In some instances, surgical intervention may be necessary. The potential gravity of these conditions and the importance of complying with voice restrictions must be understood by the patient.

DOES VOICE REST HELP LARYNGITIS?

Voice rest (absolute or partial silence) is an important therapeutic consideration in any case of laryngitis. When no professional commitments are pressing, a short course (up to a few days) of *absolute voice rest* may be considered, as it is the safest and most conservative therapeutic intervention. This means absolute silence and communication with a writing pad or other assistive, non-verbal device. The patient must be instructed not to whisper, as this may be an even more traumatic vocal activity than speaking softly. Whistling through the lips and mouthing words also require vocal fold motion and should not be permitted. Absolute voice rest is necessary only for serious vocal fold injury such as hemorrhage or vocal fold tear. Even then, it is virtually never indicated for more than 7 to 10 days. Three days are often sufficient.

In many instances of mild to moderate laryngitis, considerations of finances and reputation mitigate against an absolute recommendation of voice rest in some professional voice users. In advising performers to minimize vocal use, Dr. Norman Punt, of London, counseled: "Don't say a single word for which you are not being paid." His admonition frequently guides the ailing voice user away from pre-performance conversations and post-performance greetings.

Patients with mild to moderate laryngitis should also be instructed to speak softly (but not whisper), at a slightly higher pitch than usual and with a slightly breathy voice, to avoid excessive telephone use, and to speak with abdominal support as they would in singing. This is *relative voice rest*, and it is helpful in most cases. An urgent session with a speech-language pathologist is extremely valuable in providing guidelines to prevent voice abuse. Nevertheless, the patient must be aware that some risk is associated with performing with laryngitis, even when voice use is possible. Inflammation of the vocal folds is associated with increased capillary fragility and increased risk of worsening and permanent vocal fold injury or hemorrhage. Many factors must be considered in determining whether a given voice commitment is important enough to justify the potential long-term and possibly career ending consequences

WHAT OTHER TREATMENTS MAY BE USED FOR LARYNGITIS?

Steam inhalations deliver moisture and heat to the vocal folds and tracheobronchial tree and are often useful. Some people use nasal irrigations, which are very helpful for nasal allergies and infections and may help prevent allergens and secretions that are trapped in the nose from reaching and irritating the larynx.

Gargling has no proven efficacy in the treatment of laryngitis, but it may help prevent thrush infections in the larynx in patients who use inhaled steroids for treatment of their asthma. In these cases, gargling lightly with water after each steroid inhalation helps to prevent thrush infections of the larynx that typically occur because of the steroid deposition on the vocal folds. Gargling is probably harmful only if it involves loud, abusive vocalization as part of the gargling process.

Ultrasonic treatments, local massage, psychotherapy, and biofeedback directed at relieving anxiety and decreasing muscle tension may be helpful adjuncts to a broader therapeutic program. However, psychotherapy and biofeedback, in particular, must be supervised expertly if used at all.

Can Lung Problems Cause Voice Disorders?

Respiratory problems are especially problematic to singers, other voice professionals, and wind instrumentalists, but they may cause voice problems in anyone.

Support is essential to healthy voice production. The effects of respiratory infection are obvious and can affect the voice by direct laryngeal inflammation or by impairing breathing and support. Restrictive lung disease such as that associated with obesity may impair support by decreasing lung volume and respiratory efficiency. However, obstructive pulmonary disease such as asthma and COPD, are the most common culprits. Even mild obstructive lung disease can impair support enough to cause increased neck and tongue muscle tension and abusive voice use capable of producing vocal nodules.

This scenario occurs even with unrecognized asthma and may be difficult to diagnose unless suspected, because many such cases of asthma are exercised- or reflux-induced. Vocal performance is a form of exercise, whether the performance involves singing, giving speeches, sales, or other forms of intense voice use. Individuals with this problem will have normal pulmonary function clinically and may even have normal or nearly normal pulmonary function test findings at rest. However, as the voice is used intensively, pulmonary function decreases, effectively impairing support and resulting in compensatory abusive techniques. When suspected, this entity can be confirmed through a methacholine challenge test performed by a pulmonary (lung) specialist. In some individuals, pressure changes in the abdomen during intense or prolonged voice use can cause reflux episodes, which in turn can also trigger a mild asthma attack—this also may be diagnosed only with methacholine challenge tests.

Treatment of the underlying pulmonary disease to restore effective support is essential to resolving the vocal problem. Treating asthma is rendered more difficult in professional voice users because of the need in some patients to avoid not only inhalers but also drugs that produce even a mild tremor. The cooperation of a skilled pulmonologist specializing in asthma and sensitive to problems of performing artists is invaluable.

Do Stomach Problems or Hiatal Hernia Affect the Voice?

Gastrointestinal disorders commonly cause voice complaints. The sphincter (a one-way valve) between the stomach and esophagus is notoriously weak. In *reflux laryngitis*, stomach acid refluxes through this weak sphincter into the throat, allowing droplets of the irritating gastric acid to come in contact with the vocal folds and even to be aspirated into the lungs. Reflux may occur with or without a hiatal hernia. Common symptoms of reflux laryngitis are hoarseness, especially in the morning, prolonged vocal warm-up time, bad breath, sensation of a lump in the throat, chronic sore throat, cough, a dry or "coated" mouth, mucus or phlegm in the throat, throat tickle, and post-nasal drainage. Heartburn is frequently absent. Over time, uncontrolled reflux may cause cancer of the esophagus and/or larynx. So, this condition should be treated aggressively and conscientiously.

Physical examination of the larynx usually reveals a bright red, often slightly swollen appearance of the arytenoid mucosa and thick phlegm in the larynx, which help establish the diagnosis. A barium esophagogram with water siphonage may provide additional information but is not needed routinely. In selected cases, 24-hour pH monitoring provides the best analysis and documentation of reflux.

The mainstays of treatment are elevation of the head of the bed (so that the back is straight, but elevated), use of antacids, and avoidance of food for 3 or 4 hours before sleep. Avoidance of alcohol and coffee is also beneficial. Medications that block stomach acid secretion are also useful, including esomeprazole (Nexium), lansoprazole (Prevacid), omeprazole (Prilosec), pantoprazole (Protonix), rabeprazole (Aciphex), dexlansoprazole (Drexilant), cimetidine (Tagamet), ranitidine (Zantac), famotidine (Pepcid), nizatidine (Axid), and others.

In some cases, surgery to repair the lower esophageal sphincter and cure the reflux may be more appropriate than life-long medical management. This option has become much more attractive since the development of laparoscopic and robotic surgery, which have drastically decreased the risks associated with this operation, as well as the length of the hospital stay and recovery.

What About Hormones?

Hormones are complex, natural chemicals that affect a variety of bodily functions. *Endocrine problems* (i.e., those involving hormone-producing organs) also have marked vocal effects, primarily by causing accumulation of fluid in the superficial layer of the lamina propria, altering the vibratory characteristics. Mild *hypothyroidism* typically causes a muffled voice, slight loss of range, and vocal sluggishness. Inflammation of the thyroid from autoimmune disease (such as Hashimoto's thyroiditis), goiter, or thyroid nodules also can contribute to problems with hoarseness and vocal instability due to local effects on the laryngeal nerves.

Pregnancy, use of *oral contraceptives* (in about 5% of women), and for a few days prior to the *menstrual period*, the voice can also lose its range slightly and have a slightly muffled or raspy sound from fluid changes in the vocal folds (similar to the changes that are also occurring in the uterus). Premenstrual loss of vocal efficiency, endurance, and range is also accompanied by a propensity for vocal fold hemorrhage, which may alter the voice permanently. The use of some medications with hormonal activity can also permanently injure a voice. This is particularly true of substances that contain androgens (male hormones) as discussed earlier.

The larynx is sensitive to hormonal influences and changes within the body in both males and females. This is most apparent during *puberty*, when testosterone influences result in a lowering of the pitch of the voice in males, as a consequence of its effect on the musculature and the cartilages within the larynx. Estrogen and progesterone are the dominant sex hormones in women. The primary function of estrogen during the menstrual cycle is to build the uterine wall in preparation for ovulation and possible pregnancy; progesterone helps to stabilize this growth and stimulates the production of mucus in the uterus to aid in conception.

The levels of estrogen and progesterone change throughout the *menstrual cycle*, and their effects can be seen in the larynx as the levels rise and fall.[1] During the premenstrual period, levels of estrogen and progesterone are at their lowest. Many women report a change in the voice during the premenstrual period that is characterized by vocal fatigue, decreased range, loss of power, and loss of certain vocal harmonics.[1] Menopausal women report similar symptoms of voice change, including vocal fatigue, decreased power, loss of the high range, and loss of vocal quality.[1]

Secondary effects of elevated estrogen levels include growth of breast tissue, uterine tissue, and skeletal muscle, as well as an increase in bone density. As long as estrogen levels are high, skeletal muscles maintain their mass and tone and bones maintain their density and strength.

At *menopause*, estrogen levels decline. Menopause can occur as a result of the natural aging process, as a result of surgical removal of the ovaries, or as a result of chemical or medicinal inhibition of ovarian hormone production (such as occurs with the use of Lupron Depot® (leuprolide acetate for depot suspension) to decrease excess menstrual bleeding or as can occur with the use of some chemotherapeutic agents used to fight cancer). When estrogen levels decline, regardless of the reason, the result is a loss of muscle mass throughout the body and, thus, muscle weakness. Additionally, there is a loss of bone density, which predisposes some women, especially those with small body frames, to osteoporosis and bone fractures.

The larynx also changes with menopause. Because one of the chief functions of estrogen is in maintaining the tone and bulk of skeletal muscles, including those in the larynx, many women develop atrophy of the vocal fold muscles and a reduction in the thickness of the mucosa of the vocal fold with estrogen loss during menopause. This loss of muscle bulk of the vocal folds translates into increased vocal fatigue, decreased vocal intensity, changes in range, and changes in vocal agility. In some women, the cricoarytenoid joint loses some of its mobility, which also can affect vocal agility.[1]

How Does Hormonal Replacement Affect the Voice?

The use of hormone replacement therapy (HRT) in perimenopausal women has been a controversial subject in recent years. Following a 2002 study linking it to a slight increase in risk for breast cancer, heart disease, stroke, and blood clots in the large veins (but a decreased risk of colon cancer, osteoporosis, and hip fractures),[3] use of hormone replacement therapy fell. However, it may still be used effectively and preferentially in selected women with care and monitoring.

Many women function well vocally without hormone replacement. However, approximately 20 to 30% of menopausal women will report some symptoms of menopausal vocal syndrome, for which hormone replacement therapy has been shown to be of benefit.[1,2] In addition to the beneficial effects on *menopausal vocal syndrome*, hormone replacement therapy has been most beneficial in relieving the other symptoms of menopause, including hot flashes, emotional lability, atrophic vaginitis, sleep disorders, and osteoporosis.

Thus, the professional voice user with menopausal vocal syndrome may consider hormone replacement therapy, and she should discuss this with her physician, as well as discussing the risks as they pertain to her as an individual. Women who are healthy and have no known risk factors for stroke, heart disease, vascular disease, or breast cancer may consider hormone replacement therapy, understanding the increased risks of developing any one of these problems associated with the replacement.[3,4] Women who have a family history of stroke, heart disease, vascular disease, and breast cancer and those who have a history of these illnesses themselves probably should not take hormone replacement therapy because genetically, these women are already at increased risk for these events, and the addition of another risk factor may increase this risk further. However, this recommendation is based more on impression than on evidence-based research, and all such medical decisions must be individualized. This is especially important for young, postmenopausal singers (some women experience menopause in their 30s or even late 20s) who may be willing to accept some risks in order to try to preserve their singing careers.

One should be cautious about using *"herbal" preparations* from soy or other plant extracts as alternatives to hormone replacement therapy, as these are merely estrogens in different forms. The dosages of estrogen in these preparations are not regulated, and the safety has not been tested by the federal Food and Drug Administration (FDA). It is possible for one to ingest greater amounts of estrogen from these "herbal" preparations than from a prescription formulation that is tightly controlled by the FDA. Thus, if the goal is to minimize risk by not taking hormone replacement, then the use of over-the-counter herbal supplements made from plants that produce estrogens is not recommended by the authors.

Does Anxiety Have Anything to Do with the Voice?

When the principal cause of vocal dysfunction is anxiety, the physician can often accomplish much by assuring the patient that no organic (physical) difficulty is present and by stating the diagnosis of anxiety reaction. The patient should be counseled that anxiety-related voice disturbances are common and that recognition of anxiety as the principal problem frequently allows the disorder to be overcome.

Tranquilizers and *sedatives* are rarely necessary and are undesirable because they may interfere with fine motor control, affecting vocal performance adversely. Recently, *beta-adrenergic-blocking agents*, such as propranolol hydrochloride (e.g., Inderal®) have achieved some popularity in the treatment of pre-performance anxiety in singers and instrumentalists. Beta-blockers should not be used routinely for voice disorders and pre-performance anxiety. They have significant effects on the cardiovascular system and many potential complications, including low blood pressure, clotting disorders, depression, low blood cell counts, laryngospasm with respiratory distress, and bronchospasm. In addition, their efficacy is controversial.

If anxiety or other psychological factors are an important cause of a voice disorder, their treatment by a psychologist or psychiatrist with a special interest and training in voice problems is extremely helpful. This therapy should occur in conjunction with voice therapy.

Can Abusing the Voice Create Problems?

Voice abuse through technical dysfunction is an extremely common source of hoarseness, vocal weakness, pain, and other complaints. In some cases, voice abuse can even create structural problems, such as vocal nodules, cysts, and polyps. Now that the components of voice function are better understood, techniques have been developed to rehabilitate and train the voice in speech and singing. Such voice therapy improves breathing and abdominal support, decreases excess muscle activity in the larynx and neck, optimizes the mechanics of transglottal (through the vocal fold area) airflow, and maximizes the contributions of resonance cavities. It also teaches vocal hygiene, including techniques to eliminate voice strain and abuse, maintain hydration and mucosal function, mitigate the effects of smoke and other environmental irritants, and optimize vocal and general health.

A voice therapy team includes an otolaryngologist (ear, nose and throat doctor) specializing in voice, a speech-language pathologist specially trained in voice, a singing voice specialist with training in vocal injury and dysfunction, and when needed, an arts-medicine psychologist, psychiatrist, pulmonologist, neurologist, exercise physiologist, or other specialist. Progress is monitored not only by listening to the patient and observing the disappearance of laryngeal pathology when it is present, but also by the quantitative measurement of voice characteristics in the clinical voice laboratory. However, in some cases there are structural problems in the larynx that are correctable only with surgery.

What Structural Problems Lead to Voice Difficulties?

The edge of the vocal fold is complex and delicate. It must move smoothly and consistently. In addition to the masses described above, anything that interferes with the smooth motion of the complex layered structures of the vocal fold can cause hoarseness or other vocal problems. Vocal fold scar is particularly troublesome. It results in obliteration of the anatomic layers of the vocal fold and impairment of the normal vibration of the vocal fold. This produces hoarseness, and often breathiness, vocal strain and fatigue. Scar is a particularly challenging problem to treat effectively.

There are also many other structural abnormalities that can alter the voice. Some are discussed below. Others not discussed in this chapter include masses associated with arthritis, papillomas caused by the human papilloma virus, and many other problems that can be diagnosed by expert voice physicians.

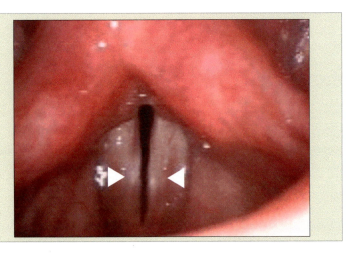

Figure 7–2. Bilateral vocal fold nodules (*arrows*).

What Are Vocal Fold Nodules?

Small, callous-like bumps on the vocal folds called nodules are caused by voice abuse (Figure 7-2). Occasionally, laryngoscopy reveals asymptomatic vocal nodules that do not appear to interfere with voice production; in such cases, the nodules need not be treated. Some famous and successful singers have had untreated vocal nodules throughout their entire careers. However, in most cases nodules cause problems with raspiness, breathiness, loss of range, and vocal fatigue. They may be due to abuse of the voice during either speaking or singing and at times occur from chronic persistent coughing.

Voice therapy always should be tried as the initial therapeutic modality and will cure the vast majority of patients, even if the nodules look firm and have been present for many months or years. In those in whom the nodules were caused by coughing, cough suppressants and medications to treat the cause of the cough are usually employed. Even in those who eventually need surgical excision of the nodules, preoperative voice therapy is essential to prevent recurrence.

Caution must be exercised in diagnosing small nodules in patients who have been speaking or singing actively. In many people, bilateral, symmetrical soft swellings at the junction of the anterior and middle thirds of the vocal folds develop after heavy voice use. No evidence suggests that people with such "physiologic swelling" are predisposed to development of vocal nodules. At present, the condition is generally considered to be within normal limits. The physiologic swelling usually disappears with 24 to 48 hours of rest from heavy voice use.

What Are Cysts?

Submucosal cysts of the vocal folds are usually caused by vocal fold trauma, meaning forceful closure of the vocal folds or laryngeal (supraglottic) hyperfunction. Cysts are formed when a mucous gland (which helps produce the lubricating mucous secretions for vocal fold vibration) within the vocal folds becomes blocked, and instead of secreting its fluid, the fluid becomes trapped inside the gland, forming a cyst (Figure 7-3). They often cause contact swelling, and some-

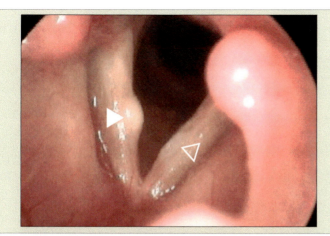

FIGURE 7–3. Subepithelial cyst on the right vocal fold (*arrow*) and a reactive mass on the left vocal fold (*open arrow*).

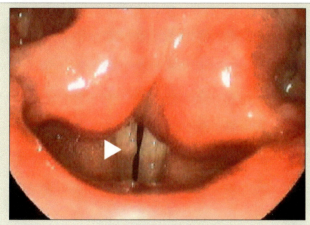

FIGURE 7–4. Right vocal fold mucosal cyst (*arrow*), with a reactive mass on the facing left vocal fold.

times nodules on the opposite vocal fold and are usually initially misdiagnosed as nodules on each side (Figure 7-4). Often, they can be differentiated from nodules by strobovideolaryngoscopy when the mass is obviously fluid-filled. They may also be suspected when the nodule on the other vocal fold resolves with voice therapy but the mass on one vocal fold persists. Cysts may also be found when surgery is performed for apparent nodules that have not resolved with voice therapy. The surgery should be performed superficially and with minimal trauma, as discussed later.

WHAT ARE POLYPS?

Many other structural lesions may appear on the vocal folds. Of course, not all respond to non-surgical therapy. Polyps are usually found on only one vocal fold, and they often have a prominent feeding blood vessel coursing along the upper surface of the vocal fold and entering the base of the polyp (Figure 7-5). The exact mechanism of formation of polyps cannot be proven in many cases, but they are thought to be formed in response to laryngeal hyperfunction in many patients. At least some polyps start as vocal fold hemorrhages (Figure 7-6).

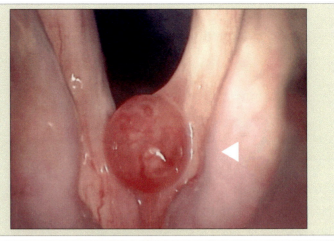

FIGURE 7–5. Left vocal fold polyp with a feeding vessel (*arrow*).

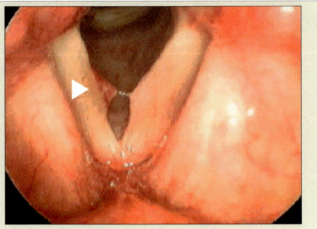

FIGURE 7–6. Hemorrhagic polyp on the right vocal fold (*arrow*) with a reactive mass on the left vocal fold.

In some cases, even sizable polyps resolve with relative voice rest and a few weeks of low-dose corticosteroid therapy. However, many require surgical removal. If polyps are not treated, they may produce contact injury on the opposite vocal fold (Figure 7-7). Voice therapy should be used to ensure good relative voice rest and prevention of abusive behavior before and after surgery. When surgery is performed, care must be taken not to damage the leading edge of the vocal fold.

What Happens if a Blood Vessel in the Vocal Folds Ruptures?

Vocal fold hemorrhage, which is bleeding into the vocal fold as a result of a ruptured blood vessel, is a potential vocal disaster (Figure 7-8). Hemorrhages resolve spontaneously in most cases, with restoration of normal voice. However, in some instances, the hematoma (collection of blood under the vocal fold mucosa) organizes and fibroses, resulting in the formation of a mass and/or scar. This alters the ability of the vocal fold to vibrate and can result in permanent hoarseness.

In specially selected cases, it may be best to avoid this problem through surgical incision and drainage of the hematoma. In all cases, vocal fold hemorrhage should

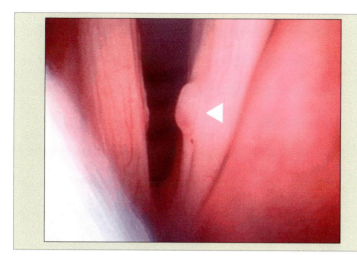

FIGURE 7-7. Left vocal fold polyp (*arrow*) with a reactive mass on the right vocal fold.

be managed with absolute voice rest until the hemorrhage has resolved and normal blood vessel integrity and vocal fold healing have occurred. Recurrent vocal fold hemorrhages are usually due to fragility of a specific blood vessel and may require surgical laser cauterization or excision of the blood vessel.

WHAT ARE THE HAZARDS OF LARYNGEAL TRAUMA?

The larynx can be injured during altercations and motor vehicle accidents. Steering wheel injuries are particularly common. Blunt anterior neck trauma may result in laryngeal fracture, dislocation of the arytenoid cartilages, hemorrhage, and airway obstruction. Late consequences, such as narrowing of the airway, may also occur (Figures 7-9 and 7-10). Laryngeal injuries are frequently seen in association with other injuries such as scalp lacerations, and the laryngeal problem is often overlooked initially, even though it may be the most serious or life-threatening injury. Hoarseness or other changes in voice quality following neck trauma should call this possibility to mind. Prompt evaluation by visualization and radiological imaging should occur. In many cases, surgery is needed.

How Can Functional or Neurologic Disorders Affect the Voice?

WHAT ABOUT VOCAL FOLD PARESIS AND PARALYSIS?

Paresis (partial weakness) and paralysis (complete weakness) may involve one or both vocal folds and one or both nerves leading to each vocal fold. When paresis or paralysis is limited to the superior laryngeal nerve, the patient loses his or her ability to control the pitch and volume of the voice, due to difficulties in stretching the vocal folds to alter the tension. Although superior laryngeal nerve paresis and paralysis involve only one muscle (the cricothyroid), the problem is often dif-

FIGURE 7–8. **A,** Left vocal fold hemorrhage and bilateral cysts (*arrows*) in a musical theater singer who had sudden voice change while singing during her menstrual period and while taking ibuprofen. **B,** After 1 week of voice rest, the hemorrhage is beginning to resolve but is still faintly present at the vibratory margin of the vocal fold. **C,** Four weeks after the hemorrhage, the changes have nearly resolved.

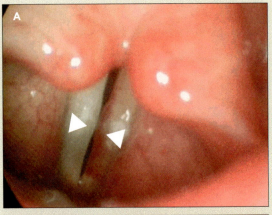
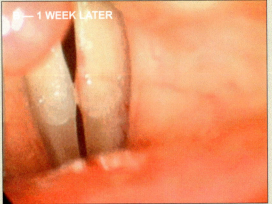
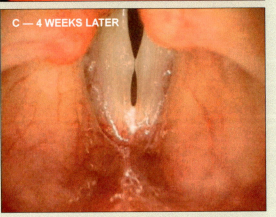

ficult to overcome. The vocal fold sags at a lower level than normal, and the patient notices difficulty in elevating pitch, controlling sustained tones, transitioning through registers, and projecting the voice. Superior laryngeal nerve paresis is caused most commonly by viral infection, especially the viruses that cause upper respiratory tract infections.

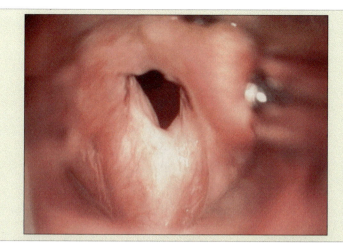

Figure 7–9. Vocal fold web (scarring) after gunshot wound to the larynx.

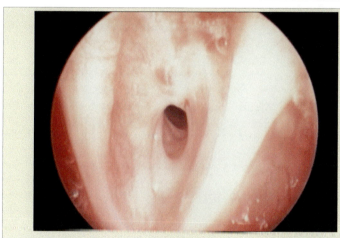

Figure 7–10. Subglottic stenosis (scarring) after endotracheal intubation.

The recurrent laryngeal nerve controls all the other intrinsic laryngeal muscles. When it is injured, the vocal fold cannot open or close well. Usually, tension is preserved and the vocal fold remains at its appropriate vertical level if the superior laryngeal nerve is not injured. If the opposite (normal) vocal fold is able to cross the midline to meet the weaker side, the vocal quality and loudness may be quite good. Compensation often occurs spontaneously during the first 6 to 12 months following nerve injury, with the weaker vocal fold moving closer to the midline. Unilateral vocal fold paralysis may be idiopathic (cause unknown), but it is also seen fairly commonly following surgical procedures of the neck such as thyroidectomy, carotid endarterectomy, anterior cervical fusion, and some chest operations.

Vocal fold paralysis and paresis should be treated initially with voice therapy. At least 6 months (and preferably 12 months) of observation are needed, unless it is absolutely certain that the nerve has been cut and destroyed, because spontaneous recovery of function is common. If voice therapy fails, vocal fold motion remains impaired, and voice quality or ability to cough is unsatisfactory to the patient, surgical treatments are generally quite satisfactory.

WHAT IS SPASMODIC DYSPHONIA?

Spasmodic dysphonia or laryngeal dystonia is a neurological disorder diagnosed in patients with specific kinds of voice interruptions. These patients may have a variety of diseases that produce the same disordered voice, which is characterized by involuntary movement in the muscles in the larynx during speech, resulting in a "spastic" sounding, strained, and occasionally breathy voice. There are some similar interruptions in vocal fluency that are occasionally incorrectly diagnosed as spasmodic dysphonia. It is important to avoid this error, because different types of dysphonia require different evaluations and treatments and have different success rates with treatment. Spasmodic dysphonia is subclassified into adductor, abductor, and mixed types.

Adductor spasmodic dysphonia is the most common and is characterized by excessive and inappropriate closure of the vocal folds during speech, producing an irregularly interrupted, effortful, strained, and staccato voice. It is generally considered neurologic in origin, and its severity varies substantially among patients and over time. In many cases, the voice may be normal or more normal during laughing, coughing, crying, or other nonvoluntary vocal activities or during singing. Adductor spasmodic dysphonia may involve the true vocal folds alone, or the false vocal folds and the supraglottis may squeeze shut as well. Because of the possibility of serious underlying neurologic dysfunction or association with other neurologic problems, as is seen in Meige's syndrome (involuntary spasms of the eyelids, facial muscles, and laryngeal muscles), a complete neurological and neurolaryngological evaluation is required. Adductor spasmodic dysphonia may also be associated with spastic torticollis (wry neck, a dystonia of the neck muscles) and/or writer's cramp (a dystonia of the hand muscles) and more generalized neurologic problems such as extrapyramidal dystonia.

Abductor spasmodic dysphonia is similar to adductor spasmodic dysphonia except that the voice is interrupted by breathy, unphonated bursts, rather than being constricted and shut off. Like adductor spasmodic dysphonia, various causes may be responsible. The abductor breaks tend to be most severe during unvoiced consonants, better during voiced consonants, and absent or least troublesome during pronunciation of vowels. Both abductor and adductor spastic dypshonia characteristically progress gradually, and both are aggravated by psychological stress, but neither is caused by stress or other psychological issues.

After a comprehensive work up to rule out treatable organic causes, treatment for spasmodic dysphonia should begin with voice therapy. Adductor spastic dysphonia is much more common, and most speech therapy and surgical techniques have been directed at treatment of this form. Unfortunately, traditional voice therapy is often not successful. Speaking on inhalation has worked well in some cases. Patients who are able to sing without spasms or interruptions but are unable to speak may benefit from singing lessons. We have used singing training as a basic approach to voice control, and then bridged the singing voice into speech.

When all other treatment modalities fail, various invasive techniques have been used. Recurrent laryngeal nerve section produces vocal fold paralysis and

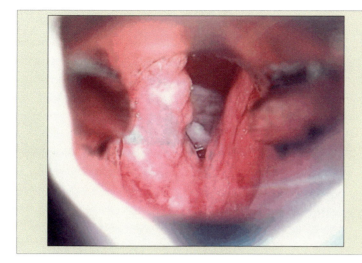

FIGURE 7–11. Laryngeal cancer affecting the right vocal fold and subglottic region.

improves spasmodic dysphonia initially in many patients. However, there is a high incidence of recurrence. We do not generally recommend this approach. Sectioning the nerve branch to only one muscle has been effective, but often short-lived.

However, the most encouraging treatment at present for patients disabled by spasmodic dysphonia is *botulinum toxin* injection. Botulinum toxin, the poison made by bacteria that cause botulism food poisoning, causes temporary paralysis of muscles in the body. Injected in small, carefully controlled amounts, it has numerous medicinal uses. Laryngeal injection is usually done with electromyographic guidance, and the technique produces temporary weakening of selected muscles in the larynx, limiting their ability to spasm and improving fluency of speech. This results in relief of the spasmodic dysphonia. However, the injections need to be repeated periodically in most patients because the effect of the botulinum toxin usually lasts only 3 to 12 months.

ARE THERE ANY OTHER NEUROLOGIC VOICE DISORDERS?

Many other neurological problems commonly cause voice abnormalities. These include myasthenia gravis, Parkinson's disease, essential tremor, and numerous other disorders. In some cases, voice abnormalities are the first symptoms of these diseases.

What About Cancer of the Vocal Folds?

Cancers of the larynx are common and are usually associated with smoking, although cancers also occur occasionally in nonsmokers (Figure 7-11). In many cases, the reason is unknown. However, it appears as if other conditions, such as chronic reflux laryngitis and laryngeal papillomas, may be important predisposing factors to the development of laryngeal cancers in both smokers and nonsmokers. Persistent hoarseness is one of the most common symptoms. Laryngeal cancers also may present with throat pain or referred ear pain.

If diagnosed early, they respond to therapy particularly well and are often curable. Treatment usually requires radiation or surgery, or a combination of the two, with or without chemotherapy in addition. It is usually possible to preserve or restore the voice, especially if the cancer is detected early. Even when the larynx is removed to treat the cancer, a prosthesis can often be placed to give a voice that is not electronic.

How Does Abdominal Surgery Affect the Voice and Vocal Performance?

As discussed in Chapter 1, the abdominal muscles contribute to abdominal support of breathing and play an important role in voice production. There are some abdominal procedures that can be performed laparoscopically, in which three to five small, 1- to 2-centimeter ($\frac{1}{2}$-inch) incisions are made in the abdomen and laparoscopes are placed into the abdominal cavity to perform the surgery with the aid of cameras, video monitors, and/or robots. Whenever possible, those who use their voice professionally and who need abdominal surgery should discuss with their surgeon or gynecologist the possibility of a laparoscopic approach. Because the laparoscopic approach does not require significant transection of abdominal muscles, it leaves most of the abdominal musculature intact and functional for use in breath support for vocal production, with a minimal need for rehabilitation following the surgery.

It is not always possible for the surgeon to use laparoscopic instruments for some abdominal surgical procedures. In these cases, incisions may be made in various locations on the abdomen to facilitate access to the organs requiring surgery. Regardless of the incision used, at least some abdominal muscles are transected (cut) with this approach. Because these muscles are cut and necessarily weakened, it is extremely important for the professional voice user to focus a significant amount of energy rehabilitating the abdominal muscles after open abdominal surgery. However, prior to beginning an abdominal rehabilitative program, consultation with and medical clearance from the surgeon who performed the surgery should be obtained to prevent injury to the surgical site and the development of hernias through the incision.

Bikini cut incisions, such as those used with abdominal hysterectomy (removal of the uterus) and cesarean section (C-section), cut through the abdominal muscles parallel to the direction of the internal oblique abdominal muscle fibers, across the fascial insertion of the external oblique abdominal muscles, and perpendicular to the rectus abdominus muscle fibers (Figure 7-12). Rehabilitation after a bikini cut approach for abdominal surgery should focus on strengthening the rectus abdominus and external oblique abdominal muscles. Standard sit-ups, crunches, and leg raises will strengthen the rectus abdominus muscle. Side bends and rotational

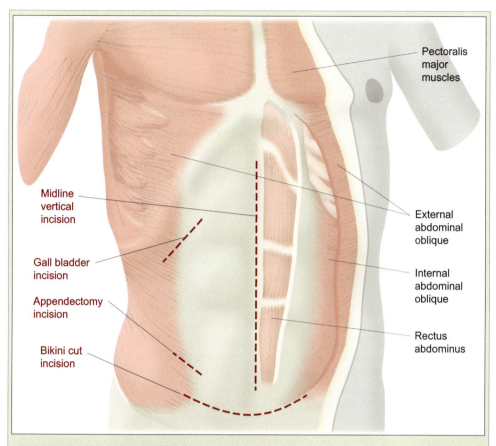

FIGURE 7–12. Locations of incisions for abdominal surgery: midline vertical incision for "open" abdominal surgery; incisions for gall bladder surgery and appendectomy; bikini incision for C-section.

abdominal exercises are good for strengthening the external oblique abdominal muscles.

A *midline vertical incision* in the abdomen (such as is done for colon surgery and many other complex abdominal surgeries) weakens the midline fascial attachment of the internal and external obliques (Figure 7-12). Following such a procedure, rehabilitation should focus on strengthening the internal and external obliques. Pilates and other exercises that focus on "core" strengthening will help with the rehabilitation of these muscles.

Incisions for *appendectomy* and *open gall bladder surgery* cut parallel to the fibers of the external obliques and transect the internal obliques at a more acute angle (Figure 7-12). Rehabilitation following these procedures should focus on strengthening the internal obliques through "core" strengthening.

During pregnancy, all of the abdominal muscles are stretched, and therefore rehabilitation after vaginal delivery should focus on strengthening all of the abdominal muscles, especially the internal and external obliques.

How Do Spine Injuries Affect Vocal Performance?

Backaches, muscle spasms, spine surgery, herniated discs, whiplash, neck pain, and other injuries to the back result in overcompensation by the uninjured side and uneven back support for the abdominal muscles. The back is the primary basis of support against which the abdominal muscles contract to help control breath support during phonation. Asymmetric or diminished back support results in an alteration in breath control and support and an inability to effectively use the abdominal muscles to their potential.

Rehabilitation from any of these injuries should be done under the supervision of a physician who specializes in spine and back injuries and with the assistance of a physical therapist. Rehabilitation should focus on re-establishing back strength, support, and symmetry and limiting pain.

Does Bedrest Affect Vocal Production?

Because of the curvature of the spine and the bony limitations of the pelvis, the abdominal organs fall toward the diaphragm while lying down, limiting lung excursion and the ability to take large breaths. Vocal production while lying on the back (termed the "supine" position) requires increased abdominal effort and a greater focus on the depth of the inhaled breath as well as the exhaled breath. Those who are on bedrest or who are bedridden can develop collapse of the lower lungs (termed atelectasis) as a result of this limited excursion of the lungs in the supine position, and they should be vigilant about remembering to take deep breaths regularly to prevent this and the subsequent development of pneumonia.

What Are the Effects of Posture, Balance, and Stance on Breathing and Voice Production?

Shifts in posture and stance affect the position of one's center of gravity, thus changing the muscles that are actively engaged in maintaining balance. For optimal breathing and voice production, posture and stance should be positioned to limit sway and contraction of the torso muscles of the back and abdomen, with the primary responsibility for balance falling on the leg muscles. Ideally, this involves standing with the feet flat on the floor, shoulder-width apart, with the knees slightly bent and the torso erect and lifted. This results in a stable stance with the center of gravity residing at about the level of the pelvis.

Standing with the feet together and knees straight shifts the center of gravity upward, and the back and abdominal muscles become more actively engaged to maintain balance. Keeping the center low frees the back and abdominal muscles to be used more effectively in breath support. In doing so, this allows the abdomen and back muscles to be used solely for breathing and breath support. This is the science behind many of the different acting, singing, and dance techniques and exercises for posture and breathing. Injuries to the feet, ankles, legs, pelvis, back, neck, or abdomen can alter the ability to adequately control breath support while standing and, if problematic, should be rehabilitated with the help of a physical therapist.

Dizziness and imbalance secondary to medications, alcohol, drugs, neuropathies, inner ear disease, and visual dysfunction result in excessive engagement of the back and abdominal muscles to help maintain balance, thus lessening the use of these muscles for breath support. Anxiety, fear, grief, and other emotions involve tension of many of the muscles in the back and the abdomen and alter the breathing pattern, which can affect the ability to control and provide sufficient breath support during vocal performance. Dizziness, other neurologic abnormalities that affect balance and stance, and psychological problems that can aggravate vocal problems should all be evaluated and treated by the appropriate medical professionals.

Summary

Numerous entities can contribute to voice problems. These include behavioral problems, such as overuse of the voice, vocal misuse (such as singing while ill or in an inappropriate register), and/or vocal abuse (such as yelling or screaming). Structural problems may include the formation of vocal fold cysts, nodules, polyps, scarring, or other lesions in the larynx. Neurologic abnormalities such as vocal fold paresis, vocal fold paralysis, and spasmodic dysphonia may also be contributing factors. Voice problems may be aggravated by illnesses involving other bodily systems, including diabetes, allergies, reflux, dizziness, psychological problems, and a myriad of other medical problems and should be addressed appropriately. Anyone experiencing difficulties with their voice should seek medical attention.

References

1. Abitbol J, Abitbol P, Abitbol B. Sex hormones and the female voice. *Journal of Voice* 1999; 13:424–446.
2. Sataloff RT, Linville SE. The effects of age on the voice. In: Sataloff RT. *Professional Voice: The Science and Art of Clinical Care*, 3rd ed. San Diego: Plural Publishing Group, Inc.; 2005: pp497–512.
3. Women's Health Initiative Investigators. Risks and benefits of estrogen plus progestin in healthy postmenopausal women: principal results from the Women's Health Initiative Randomized Controlled Trial. *JAMA* 2002; 288:321–333.
4. PEPI Investigators. Effects of estrogen or estrogen/progestin regimens on heart disease risk factors in postmenopausal women: the Postmenopausal Estrogen/Progestin Interventions Trial (PEPI). *JAMA* 1995; 273:199–208.

8

▲ What Is Reflux and How Does It Contribute to Voice Problems?

Reflux laryngitis occurs as a result of a backward flow of stomach acid and other stomach contents into the esophagus, up to the level of the larynx, where contact results in a chemical burn of the tissue lining of the larynx. This backward flow, or reflux, of stomach contents into the larynx and pharynx is referred to as *laryngopharyngeal reflux* (LPR), which in turn can cause reflux laryngitis as well as reflux pharyngitis (sore throat or tonsil inflammation), rhinitis (nasal congestion), sinusitis, and/or otitis media (middle ear inflammation or infection).

Laryngopharyngeal reflux and reflux laryngitis are different entities from gastroesophageal reflux disease (GERD) and esophagitis, although they are related. In order to fully understand this distinction, it is first necessary to understand the normal mechanisms of swallowing and emptying of the stomach, as both laryngopharyngeal reflux and GERD are disorders of these mechanisms.

Normal Swallowing and Gastric Emptying

The esophagus is the "swallowing tube" that connects the back of the throat (pharynx) to the stomach. The opening to the esophagus sits behind the larynx (Figure 8-1). At the top of the esophagus, behind the larynx, there is a ring-like muscle, the cricopharyngeal muscle (also referred to as the cricopharyngeus or *upper esophageal sphincter*), which normally is contracted or closed. This closed state allows air that is inhaled during normal breathing to go into the larynx, trachea, and lungs instead of into the esophagus and stomach.

When swallowing is initiated, the cricopharyngeus relaxes, opening the entrance to the esophagus and allowing food to pass into it. The muscles in the wall of the esophagus contract in a coordinated fashion to push the food down into

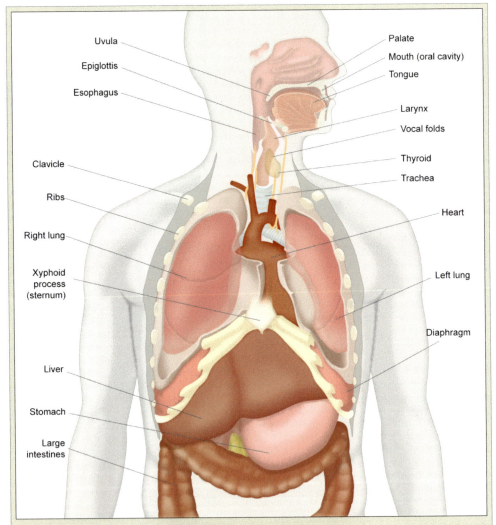

FIGURE 8–1. The respiratory system, showing the relationship between the larynx, the esophagus, the trachea, the lungs, and the diaphragm.

the stomach. At the junction of the stomach and esophagus is a sling-shaped ring of muscles in the diaphragm, called the *lower esophageal sphincter*, that is normally contracted to help keep the stomach contents in the stomach. When food in the esophagus reaches the lower esophageal sphincter (LES), it relaxes, allowing food to enter the stomach. After the swallow is complete, both the upper and lower esophageal sphincters return to their normal contracted and closed states.

When food reaches the stomach, it stimulates the stomach to release acid. The acid lowers the pH in the stomach. Enzymes from the stomach and pancreas and bile salts from the gallbladder are released into the stomach, as well. These enzymes and bile salts help in the digestion of proteins, fats, and carbohydrates. The enzymes that digest proteins are activated in the presence of an acidic environment, which is the reason that the stomach makes acid when food enters. Regardless of what kind of food is eaten, the stomach releases some acid, although certain foods stimulate the release of more acid than do others. In addition to the surge of acid secretion that occurs with eating, the stomach also has a "basal" secretion of acids; that is, there is always a baseline secretion of acid by the stomach, even when empty. The amount of acid secreted increases with meals.

In addition to the secretion of acid and the influx of enzymes and bile salts, the stomach begins to churn when food enters. The churning helps with the digestion of food, and it helps to move the food from the stomach into the intestines for further digestion and absorption of nutrients. The stomach is a sac with two openings, the gastroesophageal junction (the region of the lower esophageal sphincter) and the gastroduodenal junction (the entrance into the intestines). As stomach pressure increases, either with churning or with an increase in abdominal pressure, the contents of the stomach will flow through the opening with the least amount of resistance. As long as the lower esophageal sphincter has normal tone, this flow is directed into the intestines.

What Happens During GERD?

If the lower esophageal sphincter tone is decreased, it is less effective in blocking the flow of stomach contents into the esophagus. In such cases, when pressure in the stomach increases, the stomach contents (gastric juice) will flow through the opening of least resistance, which can be back through the lower esophageal sphincter and into the esophagus. If the sphincter has only a slight decrease in its tone, the amount of gastric juices that is allowed into the esophagus is small, as is the distance it travels up the esophagus usually. With decreasing levels of tone, more of the gastric juice can flow through the sphincter, and greater increases in stomach pressure tend to cause reflux across greater distances in the esophagus.

The esophagus is lined with "stratified epithelium," which means that the lining of the esophagus is several cell layers thick and serves as a good protective covering for the esophagus against acid injury, similar to the way in which the multiple layers of cells on the skin of the hand protect the hand from injury. Thus, small amounts of acid in the esophagus may injure the first few layers of lining cells, but will leave many layers beneath unharmed.

If the amount of acid exposure is more severe, more cell layers are injured, and injury deep to the lining tissue may occur, resulting in inflammation or esophagitis, a diagnostic hallmark of GERD. This type of injury usually produces symptoms of heartburn. GERD that is severe or that goes untreated for prolonged periods of time may result in a change in the lining tissue of the esophagus to a different cell type, a process called metaplasia, creating a condition called Barrett's esophagus, which can eventually become cancer if left untreated. Thus, everyone with symptoms of heartburn should be evaluated and treated—so should many people with other evidence of reflux (such as laryngopharyngeal reflux), even in the absence of heartburn.

What Happens During Laryngopharyngeal Reflux?

Reflux of gastric juices that travels the full length of the esophagus can reach the upper esophagus. As long as the upper esophageal sphincter has good tone, reflux will be confined to the esophagus. If tone or coordination in the upper esophageal sphincter is also decreased, then the gastric juices can escape this opening and contact the back of the larynx and the throat (pharynx and hypopharynx), a condition termed *laryngopharyngeal reflux* (LPR).

Unlike the esophagus, the larynx is lined by "pseudostratified epithelium," which usually is only one cell layer thick. This lining tissue is, thus, very sensitive to very small amounts of acid, and exposure of the larynx to acid only once or twice a week is enough to cause a significant degree of injury and inflammation in some patients. Thus, although the larynx and esophagus may be exposed to the same amount of acid, it is possible to have reflux laryngitis without any esophageal signs or symptoms of GERD, including heartburn.

Ocassionally, laryngitis may be caused by reflux that does not travel all the way up to the throat. In some patients, reflux in the lower esophagus can trigger coughing and throat clearing by stimulating the vagus nerve, which supplies fibers not only to the stomach and esophagus but also to the laryngeal nerves. However, this discussion will focus on the more common problems of laryngopharyngeal reflux caused by direct acid contact.

How Do I Know if I Have Laryngopharyngeal Reflux?

There are many symptoms of reflux laryngitis and laryngopharyngeal reflux, and any one person may have only one symptom or many. Common symptoms of laryngopharyngeal reflux are listed in Table 8-1. Although heartburn is a common symptom of GERD, it is usually not a symptom of laryngopharyngeal reflux. In fact, many people with laryngopharyngeal reflux do not experience heartburn, and many people with GERD and heartburn may not experience symptoms of laryngopharyngeal reflux. Although both GERD and laryngopharyngeal reflux may occur together in one person, it is far more common to experience either one or the other.

How is Laryngopharyngeal Reflux Diagnosed?

The diagnosis of laryngopharyngeal reflux is based on a combination of symptoms and findings in the larynx on physical examination, test results, and/or treatment response. Diagnosis is made usually by an otolaryngologist, as the larynx needs to be visualized to make the diagnosis. Although gastroenterologists and internists may place an endoscope into the mouth or nose to visualize the esophagus, many do not routinely assess the larynx and diagnose laryngopharyngeal reflux, and those

> **TABLE 8–1.** Laryngopharyngeal Reflux Symptoms and Selected Associated Conditions
>
> - Chronilc throat clearing
> - Chronic cough
> - Tickle in throat
> - Sensation of phlegm in throat
> - Sensation of swelling or "lump" in throat
> - Difficulty swallowing / food getting stuck
> - Regurgitation of swallowed food
> - Hoarseness, worse in the morning upon awakening
> - Bitter taste in mouth
> - Bad breath
> - Frequent thirst
> - "Morning voice" (prolonged vocal warm-up time)
> - Exercise-induced "asthma"
> - Intermittent periods of inability to breathe and talk (laryngospasm)
> - Awakening from sleep gasping for air
> - Dry mouth and/or throat
> - Adult-onset "asthma"
> - Sensation of post-nasal drainage
> - Sleep disturbance
> - Selected symptoms of "asthma"
> - Recurrent respiratory infections

who do are not as familiar with subtle changes in the larynx that suggest reflux disease. The larynx is typically examined by the otolaryngologist with a mirror or with a flexible or rigid laryngoscope.

Because the opening to the esophagus sits behind the arytenoid cartilages and the back of the larynx, these areas are most affected by reflux (Figure 8-2). Typically, the larynx shows signs of contact irritation and inflammation in these regions, as evidenced by the presence of redness (erythema) and swelling (edema) of the arytenoids, the interarytenoid region (the area between the arytenoids, also referred to as the posterior glottis), and the posterior cricoid region (the tissue behind the arytenoids that separates the larynx from the esophageal opening).

In severe cases, the reflux material can contact other parts of the larynx, causing erythema and edema of the vocal folds (Figure 8-3), the supraglottis (the portion of the larynx above the vocal folds) (Figure 8-4), and/or the subglottis (the portion of the larynx below the vocal folds, including the trachea). With chronic, severe acid exposure, the tissue lining the back of the larynx and/or the vocal folds may begin to produce keratin (the substance in skin that contributes to its tough, resilient nature) (Figure 8-5). Keratin is normally not present in the larynx and is produced as the body's way of protecting itself from chronic injury. This change is often referred to as keratosis or hyperkeratosis and is thought to be a precursor to the development of cancer.

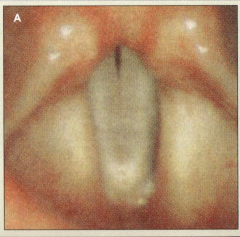
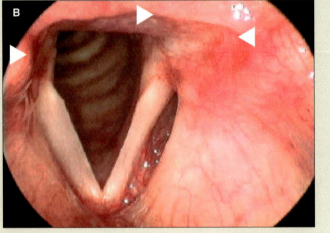

FIGURE 8–2. **A,** Normal larynx without evidence of reflux, and **B,** a larynx with reflux laryngitis, characterized by redness and swelling on and between the arytenoids (*arrows*).

Reflux laryngitis is also thought to be at least one of the factors contributing to the development of abnormal muscle use patterns in the larynx (commonly referred to as muscle tension dysphonia or laryngeal hyperfunction); nodules (see Figure 7-2 in Chapter 7), polyps (see Figures 7-5 and 7-6), and cysts (Figures 8-6) of the vocal fold; vocal process granulomas (Figure 8-7); and vocal process ulcerations. One common theory to explain these associations is that the acid burn from the reflux material in the larynx causes abnormal or decreased sensations in the larynx, similar to the way in which a burn on the finger may cause abnormal sensations there. Some of these sensations may include a throat tickle, a cough, a sensation of fullness or something stuck in the throat, dry mouth, or an altered ability to sense the positioning of the vocal folds. Hyperfunctional voice use patterns may develop from such altered sensations, which can cause increased pressure and tension on the vocal folds during speech and singing and can result in the development of vocal fold lesions.

There are few conditions that cause inflammation of the larynx in the same characteristic pattern as reflux, and laryngeal examination is usually quite effective

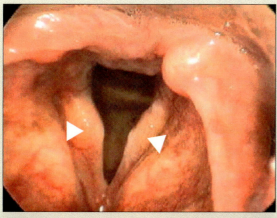

Figure 8–3. Severe polypoid edema of the vocal folds (*arrows*).

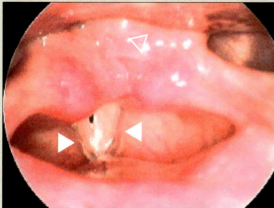

Figure 8–4. Diffuse inflammation (edema) of the larynx, involving the supraglottis, arytenoids (*arrows*), post-cricoid larynx (*open arrow*), and the vocal folds.

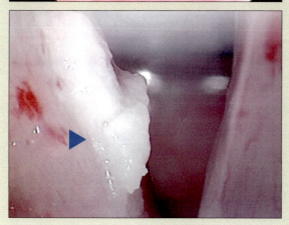

Figure 8–5. Right vocal fold hyperkeratosis (keratin on the vocal fold, *arrow*).

in detecting laryngopharyngeal reflux and reflux laryngitis. In some instances, it is also desirable to evaluate for GERD. Esophagoscopy (the endoscopic evaluation of the esophagus) may be performed to assess for esophagitis and Barrett's esophagus. However, treatment of reflux laryngitis is instituted usually based on the findings of laryngeal examination and the history.

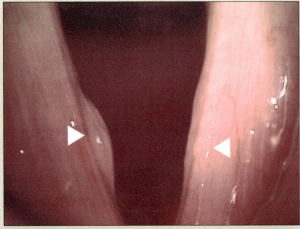

Figure 8–6. Right vocal fold cyst with overlying scar and left reactive nodule (*arrows*).

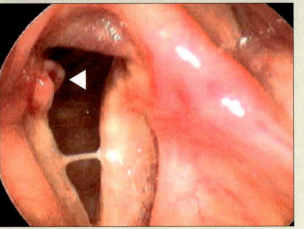

Figure 8–7. Right vocal fold granuloma (*arrow*).

Patients who do not respond well to standard treatment may require further testing, including 24-hour dual probe pH or impedance testing, esophageal manometry, esophagoscopy, and/or barium swallow. Of these studies, 24-hour dual probe impedance monitoring is the most reliable in the diagnosis of laryngopharyngeal reflux, and this test often is combined with esophageal manometry.

Esophageal Manometry

Esophageal manometry is a test in which the resting pressures of the lower esophageal sphincter, the upper esophageal sphincter, and the contracting forces of the esophagus during swallowing are measured. A thin tube with pressure sensors is placed through the nose and into the esophagus, and the exact positions of the lower esophageal sphincter and the upper esophageal sphincter are measured, as well as their respective resting pressures. In those who are prone to develop or who have laryngopharyngeal reflux, both resting pressures may be decreased, implying decreased tone or contraction at rest. However, reflux can occur even with elevated pressures.

The exact positions of the lower esophageal sphincter and the upper esophageal sphincter are determined during manometry, which allows for the correct positioning of the sensors for 24-hour impedance monitoring. Without locating the lower esophageal sphincter via manometry, the sensors will be positioned incorrectly, rendering the results of impedance testing inaccurate.

24-Hour Dual-Probe pH Testing and 24-Hour Impedance Testing

The 24-hour pH probe study had previously been used routinely and may still be helpful if 24-hour impedance testing cannot be obtained. The pH probe study only measures the presence or absence of acid in the esophagus. The impedance study measures the presence of acid, base (as can occur with bile reflux), liquid, solid, and neutral pH reflux material and, thus, is a better study for evaluating for both acid and non-acid reflux.

Impedance testing uses a monitoring system that involves the placement of a thin, plastic-coated probe through the nose and into the esophagus. The probe has two sensors on it that detect the presence of substances in the esophagus. One probe lies 5 centimeters (2 inches) above the lower esophageal sphincter, and the other probe sits close to the upper esophageal sphincter. The probe is secured to the nose with an adhesive and stays in place for 24 hours. There is a small processor that the patient wears on a belt, like a radio, that records the output of each sensor.

The patient goes home with the probe in place and is asked to resume normal daily activities. The patient is given a diary and asked to record the activities of the day, such as meals, drinking, the sensation of reflux symptoms (phlegm, throat clearing, coughing, lump in throat, etc.), exercise, singing, sexual activity, and bedtime. The processor has buttons that the patient can press to record these events when they occur. The probe is removed after 24 hours, and the information is analyzed.

The information that can be gained from the 24-hour monitoring includes the number of episodes of reflux into the lower and upper esophagus during the 24-hour period, the degree of acidity of the reflux material, the relative liquid and solid content of the reflux material, and the relationship of the reflux episodes to daily activities and to symptoms. This information can help the otolaryngologist determine whether reflux is present and symptomatic, whether anti-reflux medications are adequately controlling the pH of the reflux, and how to tailor the anti-reflux treatment to the patient's specific problem areas.

Occasionally, the results of the 24-hour monitoring are not helpful. This occurs if the patient does not happen to have any reflux episodes during the 24 hours that the monitor is in place, or if the patient's activities or diet are altered on the day of the study. For singers, actors, and public speakers, it is important to perform while the probe is in place, as reflux may occur only during singing and/or oratory speaking, which increase abdominal pressure and can cause reflux episodes when proper breath support is utilized and may not be detected otherwise.

Esophagoscopy

Esophagoscopy is the endoscopic evaluation of the esophagus by direct visualization. Esophagoscopy is most easily performed with a small endoscope that goes through the nose, with the patient awake and alert. This technique is called transnasal esophagoscopy (TNE). Esophagoscopy can also be performed with endoscopes that go through the mouth (which is also referred to as upper endoscopy or esophagogastroduodenoscopy, EGD). However, these usually require sedation or general anesthesia.

The purpose of esophagoscopy is to evaluate for signs of GERD, which may occur in 15 to 25% of those with laryngopharyngeal reflux, and especially to allow for the detection of acid-induced esophageal injuries such as esophagitis, esophageal ulcers, Barrett's esophagus, and esophageal cancer. It is an important part of the diagnostic protocol in select patients with laryngopharyngeal reflux.

Barium Swallow

During a barium swallow study, the patient is given a barium liquid to drink, and x-rays and video-recordings are taken of the patient as he or she swallows the barium liquid. The barium is seen readily on the x-ray as it travels from the mouth into the pharynx, esophagus, and stomach. If the patient has reflux during the study, it will be seen as regurgitation of the barium from the stomach into the esophagus.

If no reflux is seen, then a procedure called *barium swallow with water siphonage* may be performed. In this procedure, water is swallowed after the routine barium study has been completed. X-ray pictures and video-recordings are taken again during these maneuvers. If reflux of the barium is seen after the water is drunk, then a diagnosis of reflux is made.

The barium swallow is most helpful in diagnosing coexisting esophageal abnormalities, such as esophageal narrowing (stricture) and hiatal hernia. For these reasons, both the barium swallow and the 24-hour impedance monitoring are performed as complementary studies in some patients.

How Is Reflux Treated?

Behavioral Modification

Treatment of reflux laryngitis involves a combination of medical therapy and behavioral changes (Table 8-2). Any activity that increases the intra-abdominal pressure may exacerbate the symptoms of laryngopharyngeal reflux. Such activities may include weight-lifting, sit-ups, abdominal crunches, sexual intercourse, running, dancing, aerobics, swimming, rowing, wrestling, public speaking, acting, and singing. To minimize the effects of laryngopharyngeal reflux on the larynx and vocal performance, these activities are best performed on an empty stomach or 3 to 4 hours after meals to allow for appropriate gastric emptying. Sometimes, these activities should be preceded by use of an antacid. Similarly, one should avoid eating or drinking for at least 3 to 4 hours before lying down to sleep. The presence of food in the stomach stimulates the production of acid, making one more prone to reflux while sleeping, especially if there are snoring symptoms or if nighttime reflux has been detected during 24-hour impedance testing.

TABLE 8–2. Behavioral Modifications to Treat Reflux

- Elevate head of bed by at least 6 inches.
- Avoid exercising within 3-4 hours of eating or drinking a large quantity (more than 1 cup) of water or other liquid.
- Avoid lying down to sleep within 3-4 hours after eating.
- Avoid foods and beverages that exacerbate reflux.
- Avoid singing/public speaking/acting within 3 hours after eating or drinking large quantities (more than 1 cup) of water or other liquid.
- Lose weight.
- Avoid cigarettes and nicotine-containing products.

Elevation of the head of the bed, so that the entire bed sits at an incline, the spine is straight, and the head is at least 6 inches higher relative to the feet, also helps to minimize laryngopharyngeal reflux at night while sleeping (Figure 8-8). In this position, gravity helps to keep the stomach contents in the stomach, whereas lying flat may allow the free flow of gastric juices from the stomach into the esophagus and larynx. Sleeping on more than one or two pillows is discouraged, as high elevation of the head alone usually results in a slight flexion of the abdomen, which causes pressure on the stomach throughout the night and predisposes to reflux. If a body wedge or "reflux pillow" is used instead of elevation of the head of the bed, then a full-body wedge that extends from the head to the hips so that the back is straight should be used rather than a half-body wedge. Elevation of the head of the bed can be accomplished most easily by placing wood blocks (2x4's work well), bricks, or phone books stacked between the bed frame and the box spring mattress or under the legs at the head of the bed (Figure 8-8).

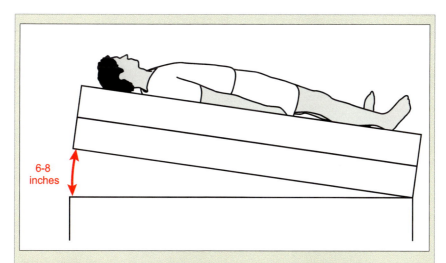

FIGURE 8–8. The head of the bed should be elevated to minimize reflux.

TABLE 8–3. Foods and Beverages that Aggravate Reflux

- Dairy products (milk, cheese, yogurt, sour cream)
- Caffeine (coffee, tea, colas, chocolate)
- Acidic foods and beverages (tomatoes, oranges, pineapple juice)
- Fatty or fried foods (pizza, French fries, fried chicken)
- Processed meats (hot dogs, sausages, bratwursts)
- Spicy foods (including onions)
- Alcoholic beverages
- Peppermint
- Licorice

Weight loss of as little as 5 pounds can also decrease the frequency of reflux episodes, probably because it usually results in less body mass in the abdominal region, thus decreasing external pressure on the stomach while sleeping.

There are several foods and food products that are known to exacerbate reflux (Table 8-3). Although it is often difficult to eliminate these foods from the diet completely, they should be consumed in moderation, if at all. Nicotine and nicotine-containing products (including cigarettes, chewing tobacco, pipes, and cigars) also increase reflux and should be avoided. The exact mechanisms by which these food products and nicotine worsen reflux is not completely understood but is believed to be through either stimulating an increased acid production in the stomach or by relaxing the lower esophageal sphincter, and in some cases by doing both.

MEDICAL MANAGEMENT OF REFLUX

The treatment of reflux consists of both behavioral modifications in the patient's lifestyle and medications. It is believed that much of the injury from reflux is also due to the effects of stomach enzymes, like pepsin, on the larynx. Pepsin becomes more active in an acidic environment, and injury in the larynx from reflux is likely due to a combination of acid and pepsin. By decreasing the amount of acid in the stomach, the activity of pepsin is decreased and the amount of acid exposure in the larynx, pharynx, and esophagus during a reflux episode is minimized. Tests that detect pepsin activity and medications that affect pepsin directly may become available in the future but are not available commercially at the present time.

The medications commonly used to treat laryngopharyngeal reflux (LPR) are proton-pump inhibitors, H2-receptor antagonists, promotility agents, and antacids (Table 8-4).

Promotility agents help to move stomach contents into the intestines faster, thus decreasing the volume of acid and stomach contents that can reflux back into the esophagus. However, because of the undesirable side effects associated with promotility agents, they are seldom used.

The other medications are used to decrease the amount of acid in the stomach (none of the medications used to treat reflux prevent reflux episodes from occurring). By decreasing the amount of acid exposure the larynx experiences from the

TABLE 8–4. Medications Used to Treat Reflux	
Proton Pump Inhibitors	**Doses Effective for LPR**
Nexium (esomeprazole)	40 mg twice daily
Prevacid (lansoprazole)	30 mg twice daily
Protonix (pantoprazole)	40 mg twice daily
Aciphex (rabeprazole)	20 mg twice daily
Prilosec/Zegrid (omeprazole)	40 mg twice daily
Dual-Release Proton Pump Inhibitor	
Dexilant (dexlansoprazole)	60 mg once daily
Adjuvant Medications to Assist in Reflux Control	
H2-Receptor Antagonists	
Zantac (ranitidine)	
Tagamet (cimetidine)	
Axid (nizatidine)	
Pepcid (famotidine)	
Promotility Agents	
Reglan (metoclopromide)	
Antacids	

reflux episodes, they may decrease the degree of injury to the larynx from each reflux occurrence. Greater amounts of acid in the larynx cause a greater degree of injury and inflammation. Usually acid suppression is needed continuously over 24 hours daily to treat laryngopharyngeal reflux and reflux laryngitis. The stomach has a basal acid secretion throughout the day that peaks in the early morning hours during sleep. In addition, surges of acid are produced each time food is eaten.

Although *H2-receptor antagonists* and *antacids* limit acid somewhat and are readily available over-the-counter, the *proton-pump inhibitors* (PPIs) clearly have superior acid suppression that provides the amount of coverage needed in those who experience laryngopharyngeal reflux. H2-receptor antagonists and antacids alone just are not strong enough.

When proton pump inhibitors are used to treat laryngopharyngeal reflux, they all need to be taken twice daily in the vast majority of patients. The only exception is dexlansoprazole, which has a built-in delayed release that gives the body a surge of medication twice a day, even though it is taken only once a day. Many of the other brands of proton pump inhibitors are marketed as a once-a-day pill, but their duration of acid suppression varies from 14 to 17 hours, and none has 24-hour acid suppression.

Treatment of laryngopharyngeal reflux requires 24-hour acid suppression and twice-daily dosing of a proton pump inhibitor, at a minimum. In some patients, even this dose is not enough, and a third or fourth daily dose of proton pump inhibitor or a bedtime dose of an H2-receptor antagonist or a specially formulated proton-pump inhibitor needs to be added. Most proton pump inhibitors work best if taken ½ to 1 hour before meals. With a twice-daily dose, this is best accomplished before breakfast and again before dinner in the evening.

Because proton pump inhibitors can decrease absorption of calcium and magnesium, individuals taking these medications should take supplemental calcium and have their primary care doctors check their magnesium levels routinely.

SURGICAL MANAGEMENT OF REFLUX

The only way to prevent reflux from occurring is to have surgery to tighten the lower esophageal sphincter. Doing so prevents gastric juices from regurgitating into the esophagus. In people in whom twice-daily proton pump inhibitor therapy is not sufficient to relieve the symptoms and damage caused by laryngopharyngeal reflux, surgical correction of the lower esophageal sphincter is the treatment of choice.

The most effective operation is called a *Nissen fundoplication*. It involves tightening of the lower esophageal sphincter by wrapping a portion of the stomach around the lower end of the esophagus, thus limiting the reflux of stomach contents into the esophagus. This procedure can be performed laparoscopically or as an "open" procedure that requires an abdominal incision. The laparoscopic approach involves operating through five small incisions in the abdomen with the guidance of telescopes. In some centers, robots are now used routinely to help with the laparascopic procedures. The open procedure involves a vertical incision along the abdominal wall and operating with direct visualization.

Other, less invasive procedures to tighten the lower esophageal sphincter by using stitches, sclerosing agents, or radiofrequency ablation through endoscopic approaches (such as the esophageal banding and the Stratta procedure) have not reached the success rates of Nissen fundoplication in the treatment of reflux. Currently, Nissen fundoplication is the only cure for reflux, with long-term success rates as high as 80 to 90%.

For professional voice users, undergoing the Nissen laparoscopic approach is preferred, as it avoids the transection of the abdominal (support) muscles that occurs with the open approach and limits significant changes in the breath support mechanism after surgery. The Nissen procedure is most effective as a treatment of reflux in those who receive partial or complete response to proton pump inhibitor therapy, but may be appropriate in other carefully selected patients.

Summary

Laryngopharyngeal reflux and reflux laryngitis are distinct entities from gastroesophageal reflux disease (GERD). In reflux laryngitis, stomach acid refluxes through the weak lower esophageal sphincter and into the throat, allowing droplets of the irritating gastric acid to come in contact with the vocal folds. Common symptoms of reflux laryngitis are hoarseness especially in the morning, prolonged vocal warm-up time, bad breath, a sensation of a lump in the throat, chronic sore throat, cough, and a dry or "coated" tongue. Typical heartburn is frequently absent. Over time, uncontrolled reflux may cause cancer of the esophagus and larynx.

Physical examination of the larynx usually reveals a bright red, often swollen appearance of the arytenoid and back of the larynx, which helps to establish the diagnosis. A barium esophagogram may provide additional information but is not needed routinely. In selected cases, 24-hour pH or impedance monitoring provides the best analysis and documentation of reflux.

The mainstays of behavioral treatment are elevation of the head of the bed (not just sleeping on pillows), use of antacids, and avoidance of food for 3 or 4 hours before sleep. Avoidance of alcohol and coffee is also beneficial. Medications that block stomach acid secretion are also useful. In some cases, surgery to repair the lower esophageal sphincter and cure the reflux may be more appropriate than lifelong medical management.

9

▲ What Does It Mean to Have a "Weak" Vocal Fold?

Vocal fold weakness is a condition where one or both of the vocal folds do not move properly. Its symptoms can range from breathiness, vocal fatigue, and decreased range, to aphonia, aspiration, and shortness of breath. It can result from a myriad of disorders that affect the nerves, muscles, or cricoarytenoid joints controlling the vocal folds. The otolaryngologist's examination is directed at determining the underlying disorder causing the vocal fold symptoms. Treatment varies depending on the cause and can include medications or surgery but almost always voice therapy.

What Are the Symptoms of Vocal Fold Weakness?

Vocal fold weakness (also referred to as paresis) is decreased or sluggish movement of the vocal folds, resulting in decreased agility of the vocal folds or, occasionally, in difficulties stretching the vocal folds to attain higher pitches of phonation.

A patient who has vocal fold weakness will likely experience problems with hoarseness, a breathy voice, and/or vocal fatigue.[1] Hoarseness is sometimes perceived because of abnormal strain in the muscles around the larynx as the patient tries to bring the vocal folds together. This excess muscle tension may sometimes result in "false vocal fold" phonation, which is a voice produced by vibrating the tissues above the vocal folds instead of vibrating the vocal folds themselves. False vocal fold phonation has a more raspy or hoarse quality than normal, true vocal fold phonation. A breathy quality is produced as a result of air escape through the incompletely closed vocal folds (Figure 9-1).

When one of the vocal folds is affected by paresis (weakness of the vocal fold due to partial injury of the laryngeal nerve) or paralysis (immobility of the vocal

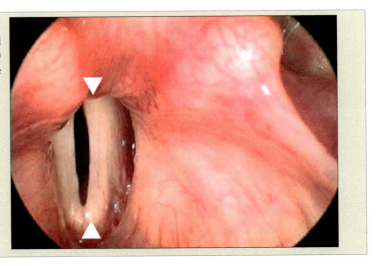

Figure 9–1. Bowed vocal fold (*arrows*) caused by paresis to the left vocal fold.

fold due to complete nerve damage), the normal vocal fold must compensate for this weakness. It does this by closing to the midline, and sometimes by closing past the midline, stretching to meet the other vocal fold. If it is unable to do this, a gap will exist between the vocal folds when the patient attempts to vocalize.

When a gap occurs between the vocal folds, the air from the lungs that is normally trapped below the vocal folds during phonation is able to leak through this gap, producing turbulence, and the sound that is perceived as breathiness and occasionally hoarseness. As air from the lungs continues to leak through the vocal folds, prolonged phonation becomes difficult because the person runs out of air on which to speak, and efforts to compensate make talking more effortful. Many describe this sensation as *vocal fatigue*. If the tensor (ability to tighten) function of the vocal folds is impaired, difficulty in changing the pitch of the voice, particularly in the extreme high range and the transition from high to mid range, may be affected as well.

One of the major functions of the vocal folds under normal circumstances is to help protect the lungs and the trachea (the windpipe that connects the larynx and the lungs) from food and liquids during swallowing (Figure 9-2). Because the back of the throat is a common passageway for food entering the esophagus and for air entering the lungs, typically the vocal folds close during swallowing to help direct food into the esophagus and away from the trachea. If the vocal folds are unable to close completely during swallowing, aspiration (the inadvertent spillage of food or liquid into the trachea and lungs) may occur.

If the sensation of the vocal folds and trachea is normal, choking or coughing should occur each time food or liquid is aspirated. If the sensory functions in the vocal folds and trachea are not working correctly, aspiration may occur without signs of choking or coughing, a phenomenon commonly referred to as "silent aspiration." Because both the superior and recurrent laryngeal nerves provide both sensory input as well as motor input into the larynx, there are some instance of vocal fold paresis or paralysis in which the sensation of the larynx is decreased as a result of the nerve injury as well.

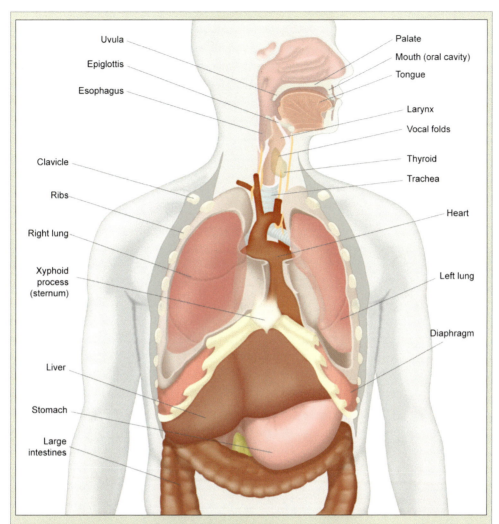

FIGURE 9–2. The respiratory system, showing the relationship between the larynx, the esophagus, the trachea, the lungs, and the diaphragm.

How Is Vocal Fold Paresis Diagnosed?

The patient who has complaints suggestive of a vocal fold paresis should be evaluated by an otolaryngologist or laryngologist. The physician will take a thorough medical history and review the individual's symptoms to help exclude other possible causes and to help narrow the potential list of problems.

After a history of the patient's problems is taken, the physician will examine the patient. The physical examination will include a complete evaluation of all of the structures of the head and neck.[2] This complete examination is performed because some disorders can affect many different regions of the head and neck, and their presence or absence helps determine optimal treatment.

Examination of the larynx is performed initially with a light and mirror. On examination with the mirror, the physician may see obvious movement disorders of the larynx. Because subtleties in movement disorders are difficult to assess with mirror examination, the otolaryngologist will almost always perform either flexible or rigid laryngoscopy, or both, for better examination of the mobility and structure of the vocal folds.[2]

Depending on the patient's complaints and the findings from the history and clinical examination, additional tests may be ordered including blood tests, laryngeal electromyography (EMG),[3] biopsy of suspect tissues, and imaging with x-rays or computed tomography.

What Causes Vocal Fold Weakness?

Vocal fold mobility can be affected by disorders of the cricoarytenoid joint, the parts of the brain and nerves that supply the larynx, or the muscles of the larynx.

CRICOARYTENOID JOINT DISORDERS

The cricoarytenoid joint can become immobile from mechanical processes in the joint space. These processes can include such entities as rheumatoid arthritis, gout, other joint disorders, infections, inflammation, trauma, arytenoid cartilage dislocation, laryngeal fracture, and surgical manipulation in the region of the arytenoid cartilages.[4-8]

Inflammation causes problems with joint mobility similar to the way in which inflammation in the fingers of the hand can cause problems with movement of the joint spaces there. Inflammation can cause injury to the joint tissues themselves and/or scarring of the tissues around the joint. When the tissues are scarred, they inhibit the ability of the cartilages to move within the joint space, resulting in decreased mobility. Dislocation or other trauma to the joint structures can also impede the normal, smooth, complex motion required in the cricoarytenoid joints for normal vocal fold movement.

MUSCLE DISORDERS

Problems with the muscles of the larynx can cause abnormal vocal fold mobility also. Laryngeal myasthenia gravis (a neuromuscular junction abnormality), amyloidosis (a general medical problem in which proteins accumulate abnormally in body tissues), edema (muscle swelling), myositis (muscle inflammation), age-related atrophy (wasting), hormonal changes, and muscular dystrophies (genetic disorders of abnormal muscle function throughout the body) are some of the disorders that may affect muscle function. The result may be vocal fold weakness or, in some cases, gaps between the vocal folds caused by insufficient muscle bulk, even if mobility is fairly good.

Myasthenia gravis is a disorder of the neuromuscular junction, the nerve-muscle interface. Myasthenia gravis can occur in multiple muscle systems throughout the body, or it can occur as an isolated entity in the larynx.[9] In myasthenia gravis, the body makes antibodies that attack the receptors on the muscle to which the neurotransmitter acetylcholine binds. Antibodies are part of the body's immune system whose main functions are to recognize foreign materials, like bacteria and viruses, and to help rid the body of these foreign materials. Occasionally, and for unknown reasons, the immune system mistakenly recognizes normal tissues as foreign, a condition referred to as an *autoimmiune disorder.*

Myasthenia gravis is an autoimmune disorder in which the antibodies attack and destroy portions of the neuromuscular junctions—these are the connections between nerves and muscles. This destruction results in an inability of the muscle to receive signals from the nerve. When this occurs, the muscle is unable to contract fully in response to nerve impulses generated when a person attempts to move the muscle, resulting in muscle weakness. Because only some neuromuscular junctions that come in contact with the abnormal antibodies are attacked in myasthenia gravis, there may be some muscles and muscle fibers that remain unaffected. This results in variability in the muscles' abilities to contract once signaled. With laryngeal myasthenia gravis, this typically is seen as fluctuating asymmetries in the ability of the vocal folds to move quickly. Patients with laryngeal myasthenia frequently complain of vocal fatigue, voice breaks, vocal instability, and inability to control the pitch and/or loudness of the voice.

Amyloidosis is a localized (affecting a single area of the body) or generalized sytemic (affecting the whole body) disorder that can involve the larynx as well as other tissues in the body, most commonly the kidneys.[6,7] In amyloidosis, an abnormal accumulation of a substance that contains antibodies is deposited in the tissues of the body. This substance is amorphous and is somewhat like gelatin in the way that it accumulates in the body's tissues. Accumulation in the larynx adds to the weight and impairs the pliability of the muscles, inhibiting their mobility.

Edema (swelling) can also cause a mass to form on the muscles of the larynx, as fluid and other substances leak out of cells and collect around muscle fibers. This can result in abnormalities in vocal fold mobility. Edema is frequently a result of inflammation. Any kind of trauma, such as infection and blunt injury (bruising) or penetrating injury to the neck and larynx, can cause edema.

Myositis is an inflammation affecting muscles alone. Immune cells accumulate in the muscle, and an inflammatory reaction, characterized by tenderness, increased blood flow, increased fluid, and increased immune cells, ensues. Myositis can occur in response to trauma or infection, but sometimes no identifiable cause is found.[14] The inflammatory fluid and the damage to the muscle membrane from the inflammation can interfere with the normal transmission of nerve impulses to the muscle, causing weakness of the vocal fold.

Muscular dystrophies are genetic disorders that are characterized by abnormal muscle metabolism (energy production). Eventually, muscle atrophy (wasting) ensues in many muscles throughout the body, including the larynx.[14] As the muscles in the larynx atrophy, they begin to lose their strength and are no longer able to move as quickly as normal or to produce the same degree of muscle tension, resulting in sluggish and bowed vocal folds. When vocal folds are bowed, they have less tension than normal, which results in a small gap between the vocal folds during closure for phonation.

With *normal aging*, there is some loss of muscle tone and bulk throughout the body, and the larynx may be involved as well. Usually this process results in bowing of the vocal folds and can produce symptoms of breathiness, decreased volume, decreased vocal agility, decreased range, and a change in habitual pitch and pitch range. For example, as women age, the pitch may lower, and as men age the pitch of the voice may rise as a result of changes in muscle mass of the vocal folds.

Because hormones play an integral role in muscle metabolism, particularly in the larynx, the voice may change with hormonal influences, too. Changes in muscle mass may be accelerated when women lose the influence of estrogen during menopause or after removal of the ovaries. Women with symptomatic voice changes due to estrogen loss may be candidates for estrogen replacement.

NERVE DISORDERS

Primary neural (nerve) disorders also may cause decreased vocal fold mobility. Injury to the superior laryngeal nerve and/or the recurrent laryngeal nerve can occur anywhere along their courses from the brain to the larynx. The term *paresis* denotes weakness and is used to describe the function of a nerve that is partially injured and partially functioning. The term *paralysis* is used to describe total absence of neural function. Injury to the vagus, superior laryngeal, and recurrent laryngeal nerves can be the result of infection, compression, metabolic abnormalities, primary nerve diseases, or direct injury.

Infection typically results from viruses such as the herpes, influenza, or parainfluenza viruses that cause the "common cold." Infection of the nerve also may result from the bacteria that cause Lyme disease or syphilis.[15,16]

Compression of the nerve can occur in response to abnormal masses that press against the nerve, such as lymphoma or tumors in the head, neck, or chest.[10] Aneurysms, which are abnormal balloon-like dilatations of the blood vessels, may also enlarge and compress the nerves. Compression also can occur during surgery as a result of the endotracheal tubes that sits in the larynx during general anesthesia or from surgical instruments used to move the larynx out of the way during spine or carotid artery surgeries, for example.

Direct injury to the nerve may occur during surgery or as a result of penetrating or blunt trauma to the neck, chest, or skull base. Depending upon how much injury is caused, each of these mechanisms can cause paresis or paralysis of the nerves that supply the larynx.

Metabolic abnormalities that can cause disorders in the nerves include diabetes mellitus and thyroid hormone abnormalities, among many other disorders. The exact mechanism by which *thyroid hormone* abnormalities cause nerve dysfunction is not fully understood, but it usually reverses once the abnormality is corrected, particularly if the treatment is started fairly early after onset of the problem.[18-20]

Diabetes mellitus is thought to cause nerve dysfunction through its effects on blood flow to the nerves. Diabetes causes long-term system-wide nerve problems because it results in the abnormal accumulation of glucose and its metabolites in the smaller vessels that supply the nerves, which eventually block the vessel lumen.[15] When the blood supply to the nerves is diminished, the nerves begin to lose their function. Damage caused by diabetes mellitus is usually irreversible.

There are also many problems that affect nerves directly. For example, *multiple sclerosis* causes damage to the insulation around nerve fibers, slowing conduction of electrical signals along the nerve. Heavy metals such as *lead* and *mercury* can produce nerve damage, and a variety of other disorders may alter nerve function and, hence, vocal fold movement.

Compression, infection, and nerve injury cause nerve dysfunction as a result of inflammation of the protective sheath that surrounds the nerve or as a result of disruption of nerve fibers or of the ability of signals to flow along the nerve. The structure of the nerve within this sheath is similar to the structure of a sausage within its casing. The nerve's protective sheath (myelin) wraps around the length of the nerve. When the sheath becomes inflamed, it swells. This swelling decreases the diameter within the sheath and impinges on the nerve that it encases. As this swelling squeezes the nerve, it becomes more difficult for electrical impulses to pass through, which results in weakness of the muscles innervated (fed) by the nerve. As long as the constriction is not severe and the nerve remains intact, the function of the nerve will eventually return as the swelling subsides.

If swelling is severe, it may completely constrict the nerve and cause the part of the nerve with the most severe constriction to die. If this occurs, as long as the sheath remains intact, the nerve will regenerate when the swelling decreases, and it will reconnect with the other intact end of the nerve inside of the sheath.

Each nerve within a nerve sheath contains hundreds of nerve fibers. When *regeneration* occurs, some of the fibers may misconnect and connect with neighboring nerve fibers within the nerve sheath. This misconnection results in abnormal movement, called *synkinesis*. When synkinesis occurs, impulses that the brain tries to send to one muscle may be directed through this misconnection to another muscle, and simultaneous movements occur.

For instance, the recurrent laryngeal nerve innervates both the posterior cricoarytenoid muscle (whichopens the vocal folds) and the thyroarytenoid muscle (which closes the vocal folds). If the recurrent laryngeal nerve is injured and synkinesis occurs, the posterior cricoarytenoid muscle may be reinnervated by nerve fibers that originally innervated the thyroarytenoid muscle. Normally, when the brain signals the thyroarytenoid muscle to contract for speech, it signals the posterior cricoarytenoid muscle to relax so that the vocal folds can come together. After synkinesis, the signal from the brain to the thyroarytenoid muscle may be rerouted to the posterior cricoarytenoid muscle via this misconnection. When the person tries to speak, the posterior cricoarytenoid muscles will contract, opening the vocal folds and causing a breathy voice.

If the nerve is severed during surgery or as the result of neck trauma, paralysis of the muscles innervated by the nerve will result. Unless the nerves are surgically reconnected (and sometimes even if they are), reinnervation is unlikely to occur spontaneously and permanent paralysis will ensue.

In general, the absence of innervation results in muscle atrophy and degeneration. If surgical reinnervation is performed, it likely will result in synkinesis for similar reasons as explained above. Even with synkinesis, however, the neural input received by the muscle usually is enough for the muscle to maintain its tone and avoid atrophy.

How Are the Disorders Treated?

Vocal fold paresis can be treated effectively for many patients using voice therapy. Expert therapy strengthens weakened vocal fold muscles. If the weakness is severe and/or therapy is not successful, surgery can be performed to bring the vocal folds closer together, closing the gap caused by vocal fold laxity due to nerve dysfunction.

Summary

Vocal fold weakness can result from a myriad of disorders of the nerves, muscles, or cricoarytenoid joint. Vocal fold weakness may manifest with symptoms that range from breathiness, vocal fatigue, and decreased range, to aphonia, aspiration, and shortness of breath. Comprehensive clinical examination, followed by laryngeal electromyography, imaging studies, biopsies, and laboratory studies as needed, may aid in determining the causes of the disorders. Management of vocal fold weakness varies depending upon the cause and can include medical, surgical, and/or rehabilitative voice therapies, but optimal treatment usually requires meticulous, systematic, sophisticated evaluation, and interdisciplinary voice team treatment.

References

1. Dursun G, Sataloff RT, Spiegel JR, Mandel S, Heuer RJ, Rosen DC. Superior laryngeal nerve paresis and paralysis. *Journal of Voice* 1996; 10:206–211.
2. Sataloff RT, Spiegel JR, Hawkshaw MJ. Strobovideolaryngoscopy: results and clinical value. *Annals of Otology Rhinology and Laryngology* 1991; 100:725–727.
3. Sataloff RT, Mandel S, Manon-Espaillat R, Heman-Ackah YD, Abaza M. *Laryngeal Electromyography*, 2nd ed. San Diego, CA: Plural Publishing Inc.; 2006.
4. Bridger MW, Jahn AF, van Vostrand AW. Laryngeal rheumatoid arthritis. *Laryngoscope* 1980; 90:296–303.
5. Lawry GV, Finerman ML, Hanafee WN, Mancuso AA, Fan PT, Bluestone R. Laryngeal involvement in rheumatoid arthritis: a clinical, laryngoscopic, and computerized tomographic study. *Arthritis and Rheumatology* 1984; 27:873–882.
6. Goodman M, Montgomery W, Minette L. Pathologic findings in gouty cricoarytenoid arthritis. *Archives of Otolaryngology* 1976; 102:27–29.
7. Paulsen FP, Jungmann K, Tillmann BN. The cricoarytenoid joint capsule and its relevance to

endotracheal intubation. *Anesthesia & Analgesia* 2000; 90:180–185.
8. Sataloff RT, Bough ID, Spiegel JR. Arytenoid dislocation: diagnosis and treatment. *Laryngoscope* 1994; 104:1353–1361.
9. Nieman RF, Mountjoy JR, Allen EL. Myasthenia gravis focal to the larynx: report of a case. *Archives of Otolaryngology* 1975; 101:569–570.
10. Hellquist H, Olofsson J, Sokjer H, et al. Amyloidosis of the larynx. *Acta Otolaryngologica* 1979; 88:443–450.
11. Berg AM, Troxler RF, Grillone G, et al. Localized amyloidosis of the larynx: evidence for light chain composition. *Annals of Otology Rhinology and Laryngology* 1993; 102:884–889.
12. Bennett JD Chowdhury CR. Primary amyloidosis of the larynx. *Journal of Laryngology and Otology* 1994; 108:339–340.
13. Lewis JE, Olsen KD, Kurtin PJ, et al. Laryngeal amyloidosis: a clinicopathologic and immunohistochemical review. *Otolaryngology Head Neck Surgery* 1992; 106:372–377.
14. Mandel S, Manon-Espaillat R, Patterson SD, Sataloff RT. Laryngeal EMG: electromyographic evaluation of vocal fold disorders. *Journal of Singing* 1998; 55:43–48.
15. Rabkin R. Paralysis of the larynx due to central nervous system syphilis. *Eye Ear Nose Throat Monthly* 1963; 42:53.
16. Neuschaefer-Rube C, Haase G, Angerstein W, Kremer B. Einseitige rekurrensparese bei verdacht auf Lyme-borreliose [Unilateral recurrent nerve paralysis in suspected Lyme borreliosis]. *HNO* 1995; 43:188–190.
17. Heman-Ackah YD, Batory M. Determining the cause of mild vocal fold hypomobility. *Journal of Voice* 2003; 17(4):579–588.
18. McComas AJ, Sica RE, McNabb R, et al. Neuropathy in thyrotoxicosis. *New England Journal of Medicine* 1973; 289:219–221.
19. Misiunas A, Niepomniszcze H, Ravera B, et al. Peripheral neuropathy in subclinical hypothyroidism. *Thyroid* 1995; 5:283–286.
20. Torres CF, Moxley RT. Hypothyroid neuropathy and myopathy: clinical and electrodiagnostic longitudinal findings. *Journal of Neurology* 1990; 237:271–274.

10 What Are Non-Surgical Options for Treating Voice Problems?

For many people with voice difficulties, there is usually more than one medical condition that is contributing to the voice problem. A thorough physical examination will help to elucidate which problems, in particular, are contributing factors, and proper treatment will often offer significant benefit.

What Drugs Are Used for Voice Dysfunction?

ANTIBIOTICS

When antibiotics are used to treat vocal dysfunction due to infection, high doses to achieve therapeutic blood levels rapidly are recommended, and a full course (usually 7 to 14 days) should be administered. Starting treatment with an intramuscular injection may be helpful if there is time pressure.

ANTI-REFLUX MEDICATIONS

When reflux is a contributing factor to the voice complaint, anti-reflux medications, as discussed in Chapter 8, can be helpful. Although many reflux medications are available over-the-counter, it is always advisable to have a laryngeal examination prior to beginning any of these preparations, as there may be other issues contributing to the voice problem that can be masked by improvement in the reflux component of the voice disorder.

Antihistamines and Mucolytics

Antihistamines—such as loratidine (brandname Claritin®), certirizine (Zyrtec®), levocertirizine (Xyzal®), fexofenadine (Allegra®), diphenhydramine (Benadryl®), chlorpheniramine (Chlor-Trimeton®), and triprolidine (Actifed®)—may be used to treat allergies. However, because they tend to cause dryness and are frequently combined with decongestants that further reduce and thicken mucosal secretions, they may reduce lubrication to the point of producing a dry cough. This dryness may be more harmful than the allergic condition itself.

Antihistamines with less severe side effects (such as loratidine, certirizine, levocertirizine, or fexofenadine) in small doses should be tried between voice commitments. Again, they should generally not be used for the first time immediately before performances if the vocalist has had no previous experience with them.

The adverse effects of antihistamines may be counteracted to some extent with mucolytic expectorants that help to liquefy thick mucus and increase the output of thin respiratory tract secretions. Guaifenesin, the most commonly prescribed mucolytic, thins and increases secretions. Mucinex® is one of the convenient and most effective preparations of guaifenesin available and can be purchased over-the-counter. Thise drug is relatively harmless and may be very helpful to patients who experience thick secretions, frequent throat clearing, or "postnasal drip."

Steroids are a highly effective alternative to antihistamines for treating acute allergic attack immediately prior to a voice commitment, but must be used sparingly. Singulair® (montelukast) is an allergy medication that works directly on the inflammatory cells that cause allergic reactions. Because it is not an antihistamine, it does not have drying effects on the vocal folds and is the preferred allergy medication for professional singers.

Steroids

Corticosteroids are potent anti-inflammatory agents and may be helpful in managing acute inflammatory laryngitis. Although many laryngologists recommend using steroids in low doses (methylprednisone 10 mg), the authors have found higher doses for short periods to be more effective. Depending on the indication, common dosages include prednisone 60 mg or dexamethasone 6 to 10 mg intramuscularly once, or a similar starting dose orally tapered over 3 to 6 days.

Regimens such as a methylprednisolone (Medrol®) dose pack may also be used. If there is the possibility that the inflammation may be of infectious origin, antibiotic coverage is generally recommended in addition to the steroids. Care must be taken not to prescribe steroids excessively.

Anabolic steroids, which have received so much attention because of their abuse by athletics, are not used for voice treatment and may masculinize the voice.

Diuretics

In the premenstrual period, altered female hormone levels of estrogen and progesterone occur and can cause an associated increase in circulating antidiuretic hormone levels. Antidiuretic hormone causes fluid retention in the superficial layer of the lamina propria (Reinke's space) of the vocal fold and can cause temporary deepening of the voice, voice breaks, difficulties with register transitions and, in some cases, raspiness. This fluid accumulation is attached to proteins in Reinke's space and does not respond effectively to diuretics, which are sometimes prescribed by gynecologists to help lessen the abdominal fluid retention that also occurs during the premenstrual and menstrual periods.

In the larynx, these diuretics are not only ineffective, they are also counterproductive, having the undesirable side effect of dehydrating the patient and, thus, the vocal folds. Dehydration decreases vocal fold lubrication and predisposes the vocalist to vocal fold tears, hemorrhages, edema, and nodule/scar formation. Diuretics have no place in the treatment of premenstrual voice disorders. If they are used for other medical reasons, their vocal effects should be monitored closely.

ASPIRIN AND NON-STEROIDAL ANTI-INFLAMMATORY DRUGS (NSAIDs)

Aspirin and other non-steroidal anti-inflammatory drugs (for example, ibuprofen [brandnames Motrin® and Advil®] and naproxen [brandnames Naprosyn® and Aleve®]) frequently have been prescribed or taken for the relief of minor aches and pains, including throat and laryngeal irritations. However, both aspirin and NSAIDs cause decreased ability of the blood to form a clot, which predisposes to bleeding and hemorrhage, especially in vocal folds traumatized by excessive voice use in cases of vocal dysfunction. Vocal fold hemorrhage can be devastating to a professional voice user, and people who depend on extensive voice use should avoid aspirin and NSAID products altogether, unless they are absolutely necessary for the treatment of specific medical conditions.

Acetaminophen is the best substitute, as it has no adverse effect on the clotting mechanism. Care should be taken in taking acetaminophen with alcohol, as the combination can have deleterious effects on the liver.

Pain is an important protective physiologic function. Masking pain by taking pain medications, topical analgesic sprays, or steroids risks incurring grave vocal damage that may be unrecognized until after the medication wears off. If a patient requires analgesics or topical anesthetics to alleviate laryngeal discomfort, the laryngitis is severe enough to warrant canceling a vocal performance.

If the analgesic is for headache or some other discomfort not intimately associated with voice production, symptomatic treatment should be discouraged until demanding vocal commitments have been completed. In these instances, the ability to sense pain or other abnormal sensations in the larynx can be altered by the pain medication, which can also predispose to serious vocal injury.

SPRAYS AND INHALANTS

The use of analgesic topical sprays in the throat and mouth is extremely dangerous and should be avoided. Diphenhydramine hydrocholoride (Benadryl®), 0.5% in distilled water, delivered to the larynx as a mist is a formerly popular treatment that may be helpful for its vasoconstrictive properties, but it is also dangerous because of its analgesic effect. It should not be used.

Other topical vasoconstrictors that do not contain analgesics may be beneficial in selected cases. Oxymetazoline hydrochloride (Afrin®), a nasal spray, is particularly helpful in rare, extreme circumstances. Propylene glycol 5% in a physiologically balanced salt solution may be delivered by large-particle mist and can provide helpful lubrication shortly before performance, particularly in cases of laryngitis sicca (dry throat) after air travel or in dry climates. Such treatment is harmless and may also provide a beneficial placebo effect.

Water or saline solution delivered via a vaporizer or steam generator is frequently effective and sufficient. This therapy should be augmented by oral hydration (that is, drinking lots of water), which is the mainstay of treatment for dehydration. Voice users should monitor their state of hydration by observing their urine color. The more pale the urine, the better the state of hydration. A dark or amber-colored urine implies that the body could use more water.

What Else Can Be Done to Help a Person with Voice Problems?

Voice lessons given by an expert teacher are invaluable for singers and even many non-singers with voice problems. When technical dysfunction is suspected or identified, the singer should be referred to the teacher. Even when an obvious physical abnormality is present, referral to a voice teacher is appropriate, especially for younger singers. Numerous "tricks of the trade" permit a singer to safely overcome some of the disabilities of mild illness safely. If a singer plans to proceed with a performance during an illness, he or she should not cancel voice lessons as part of the relative voice rest regimen; rather, a short lesson to assure optimum technique is extremely useful.

For non-singers, training with a knowledgeable singing teacher under medical supervision is often extremely helpful for those with voice problems. In conjunction with therapy under the direction of a certified licensed speech-language pathologist, appropriate singing lessons can provide the patient with many of the athletic skills and "tricks" used by performers to build and enhance the voice. Once singing skills are mastered even at a beginner level, the demands of routine speech become trivial by comparison.

Special skills can be refined even further with the help of an acting voice trainer, who may also be part of a medical voice team. Such training is invaluable for any public speaker, teacher, salesperson, or anyone else who cares to optimize his or her communication skills.

What About Voice Therapy?

Voice therapy is generally provided under the supervision of a certified, licensed, speech-language pathologist (SLP). An SLP usually has a master's degree or PhD and is a trained health professional. However, an individual SLP's training may or may not include skills in the management of voice disorders. SLPs care for many other problems, such as swallowing therapy following strokes. Hence, it is important to find an SLP with special interests, training, and expertise in voice problems.

Therapy generally begins with procedures to analyze the voice problem. The analysis process includes subjective assessment by the SLP, as the patient speaks and performs a variety of vocal tasks. Objective voice analysis is also extremely helpful and is available in more sophisticated centers. The process uses a variety of instruments to measure, quantify, and analyze various aspects of voice production. The information obtained from voice therapy can be extremely helpful when designing voice therapy that accomplishes the desired goals optimally and quickly.

Voice therapy is really a form of physical therapy for the voice. It usually involves exercises that help a person eliminate abusive vocal habits, relax unnecessarily tense muscles, and learn to use the voice efficiently and effectively. Patients need to practice between therapy sessions in order to achieve the desired results. Therapy generally results in improvement in vocal quality, ease, and endurance. In some cases, it may also produce resolution (cure) of structural abnormalities, such as nodules.

Voice therapy is enhanced often when given in combination with retraining provided by an expert singing voice specialist and/or acting voice specialist.

Summary

Because the development of voice difficulties usually has multiple causative factors, treatment is often multifactorial as well. Treatment of allergies, infections, nasal congestion, reflux, and other medical conditions will usually hasten recovery and aid voice therapy. Voice therapy with a qualified SLP in conjunction with singing therapy can provide the individual with techniques to hasten vocal recovery and prevent further injury.

11

▲ When Is Voice Surgery Indicated?

Although all reasonable efforts should be made to avoid operative intervention, there are times when surgery is appropriate and necessary. Ultimately, the decision depends on a risk-benefit analysis. For example, if a professional voice user is unable to continue his or her career and surgery may restore vocal function, surgery certainly should not be withheld. However, the patient must understand the risks clearly. Anytime one operates on the vocal fold, there is a chance of making the voice permanently worse. All patients with voice difficulties must clearly recognize this risk and must consider it an acceptable risk in light of ongoing vocal problems.

Surgery can cure many voice problems, but it may also result in complications that worsen the voice. Scar tissue occurs in response to trauma, including surgery. If scar tissue replaces the normal anatomic layers, the vocal fold becomes stiff and adynamic (non-vibrating). This results in asymmetric, irregular vibration with air turbulence that we hear as hoarseness, and/or incomplete vocal fold closure allowing air escape which makes the voice sound breathy. Such a vocal fold may look normal on traditional examination, but it will be seen as abnormal under stroboscopic light.

Conveniently, most benign pathology (nodules, polyps, cysts, etc.) is superficial. Consequently, surgical techniques have been developed to permit removal of lesions from the epithelium or superficial layer of the lamina propria without disruption of the intermediate or deeper layers in most cases, thus minimizing the risk of scarring and worsening of the voice. All of these delicate microsurgical techniques are now commonly referred to as *phonomicrosurgery*.

Singing teachers and speech-language pathologists working with the patient are called on routinely to participate in the decision making process. They also should understand the possible considerations involved in determining whether surgery is necessary and the adjunctive treatments that accompany surgery in state-of-the-art voice care centers.

Is Pre-operative Voice Therapy Necessary?

Voice surgery should nearly always be preceded by a therapeutic trial of voice therapy. There are rare exceptions, such as acute vocal fold hemorrhage that fails to resolve, but in the vast majority of patients, preoperative voice therapy is integral to successful surgery. In some cases, it obviates the need for surgery. In others in which voice therapy alone may prove insufficient, it helps the patient and health care team recognize that surgery is justified and is an unavoidable course on the road to voice improvement. In all instances, the best postoperative voice therapy begins as good preoperative voice therapy.

The preoperative assessment and therapeutic process should also take into account the patient's psychological condition. The psychologist or psychiatrist is an important part of the voice care team and should be involved whenever appropriate. It is essential to address the patient's fears, problems, and concerns; to educate the patient; and to have the patient fully prepared to comply with, and actively assist in, the therapeutic process. Surgeons must remember that the patient is the most important member of the voice care team.

How Is the Timing of Surgery Decided?

The timing of voice surgery is also important to the therapeutic outcome. Many factors must be taken into account, including the ability to schedule preoperative therapy, the menstrual cycle (particularly in patients who suffer from premenstrual voice changes), the use of medications (such as aspirin and other anticoagulants), timing of severe seasonal allergy symptoms, control of reflux, and other medical conditions. When selected nonsurgical treatments fail and when a patient remains sufficiently symptomatic to warrant the surgical risks in the opinion of the patient, voice therapist, and laryngologist, meticulous microsurgery usually results in voice improvement.

What Conditions Require Surgery?

VOCAL FOLD NODULES

Vocal nodules are caused ordinarily by chronic voice abuse or misuse. Normally, they are present on both vocal folds, are fairly symmetrical in size and appearance, and typically are solid, benign masses near the junctions of the front and middle thirds of the vocal folds (Figure 11-1). Because this region of the vocal folds is receiving most of the impact from forceful vocal fold closure, this region is often referred to as the "striking zone." Occasionally, laryngoscopy reveals asymptomatic vocal fold nodules, or in other words, they do not interfere with voice production and should not be removed.

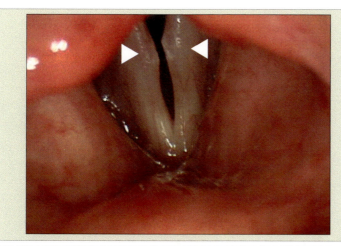

Figure 11–1. Bilateral vocal fold nodules (*arrows*).

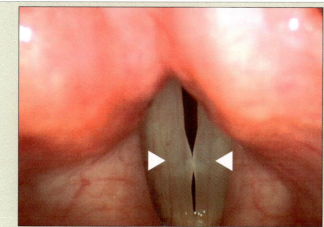

Figure 11–2. Bilateral vocal fold cysts (*arrows*) that could be mistaken for nodules on low-magnification examination of the larynx.

Most nodules respond to expert voice therapy. When they fail to respond, an incorrect diagnosis should be suspected first. Cysts may "masquerade" as nodules—for example, they both tend to occur in the same location on the vocal fold (Figure 11-2). If a patient has complied with appropriate voice therapy for 6 to 8 weeks, symptoms persist, and on follow-up strobovideolaryngoscopy there is no substantial visual improvement in the appearance (size) of vocal fold nodules, surgery may be appropriate.

Vocal Fold Cysts

Vocal fold cysts are generally unilateral (on one vocal fold), although they often cause contact swelling on the contralateral (opposite) side (Figure 11-3). They may also be bilateral. Cysts are fluid-filled, whereas nodules are solid. Cysts are frequently misdiagnosed as vocal fold nodules initially, although this error can be avoided through the use of strobovideolaryngoscopy with sufficient magnification. Voice therapy should be tried, especially to help resolve contralateral contact swelling. Symptomatic cysts often require surgery.

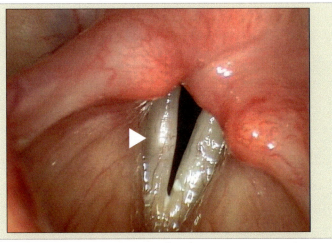

Figure 11–3. Right vocal intracordal cyst (*arrow*).

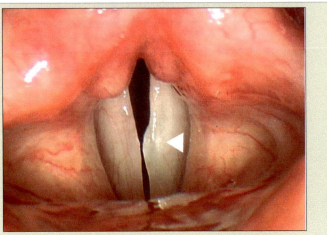

Figure 11–4. Left vocal fold polyp (*arrow*).

VOCAL FOLD POLYPS

Vocal fold polyps are usually unilateral, and they often have a prominent feeding blood vessel coursing along the superior surface of the vocal fold and entering the base of the polyp (Figure 11-4). Polyps may be loose, gelatinous masses, or more solid. Contributing factors such as voice abuse and reflux should be controlled. Voice therapy and oral steroids may be tried. However, most polyps eventually require surgical removal.

REINKE'S EDEMA

Reinke's edema is characterized by gelatinous fluid in the area just under the surface of the vocal folds (Reinke's space), creating a typical floppy, "elephant ear," or polypoid appearance of the vocal fold (Figure 11-5). It is most commonly associated with smoking, but voice abuse, reflux, and hypothyroidism may also contribute. This condition causes a low-pitched, gravelly voice.

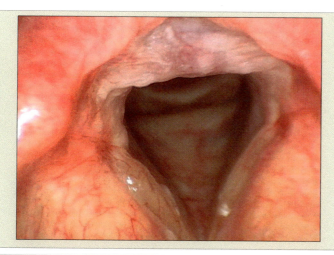

Figure 11–5. Bilateral vocal fold Reinke's edema.

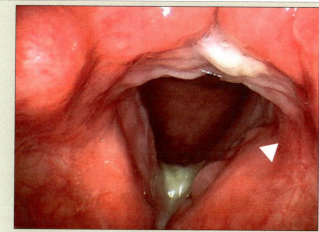

Figure 11–6. Left false vocal fold granuloma (*arrow*) from reflux.

If the patient is disturbed by his or her voice quality and wishes to have voice improvement, surgery is usually effective. It should be noted, however, that many of these patients are happy with their voice and do not want to change or improve its quality. Unless there is any suspicion of cancer (which can occur in patients with a history of smoking, alcohol or drug use), surgeons should abide by the patient's wishes.

Granuloma

Granulomas are the laryngeal equivalent of "scabs" that form in response to repeated trauma on the portion of the vocal fold that connects to the arytenoid cartilage. They may occur on one or both vocal folds. The vast majority are due to a combination of laryngeal hyperfunction and laryngopharyngeal reflux. Occasionally, the trauma from intubation during surgery or a hospitalization may contribute to granulomas formation. Voice abuse is also a common factor and may be the primary or sole cause (Figure 11-6). Granulomas must also be distinguished from other condi-

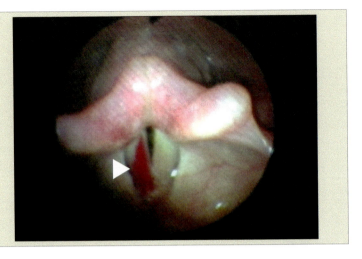

FIGURE 11–7. Right vocal fold hemorrhage (*arrow*).

tions that may present with a similar appearance, including cancer, tuberculosis, tumors, and others.

When granulomas do not resolve promptly through medical means and voice therapy, surgery is appropriate. Botulinum toxin (Botox®) is used occasionally, as well. Botox temporarily weakens a vocal fold, helping to prevent further injury from harsh contact during vocal fold closure and is helpful when granulomas are caused by severe voice abuse and in selected other cases.

VOCAL FOLD HEMORRHAGE

Hemorrhage (bleeding) into the vocal folds usually resolves spontaneously, but scarring (fibrosis) may develop in some cases (Figure 11-7). If there is a large hematoma (collection of blood inside the tissue) involving a vocal fold, and if the hematoma does not flatten within 24 to 48 hours, surgical evacuation should be considered.

SULCUS VOCALIS

Sulcus vocalis is a groove in the membranous portion of the vocal fold, usually extending throughout its length (Figure 11-8). In a true sulcus, the lining tissue invaginates through the superficial layer of the lamina propria (Reinke's space) and adheres to the vocal ligament. Sulcus vocalis can be present at birth or can be acquired from trauma, surgery, or vocal fold masses. When it is present and causing voice symptoms that are unacceptable to the patient, surgery may be considered. In these cases, the patient must be warned that it is reasonable to expect improvement in vocal quality, but not perfection.

LARYNGEAL WEBS

Webs, which are bands of scar connecting the vocal folds, may be congenital or acquired following trauma or surgery (Figure 11-9). They may be treated surgically if they are symptomatic. However, many patients with webs have satisfactory

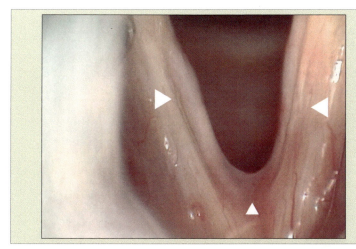

FIGURE 11–8. Bilateral sulcus vocalis (*arrows*) and small glottic web (*small arrow, bottom*).

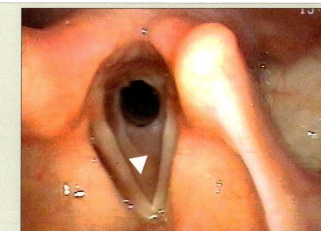

FIGURE 11–9. Laryngeal web (*arrow*).

voices, even for professional purposes. It must be remembered that resection of the web may restore normal vocal fold length, but the region of the web may remain stiff. In such cases, the postoperative voice may be worse. Surgery on asymptomatic or minimally symptomatic webs should be performed only with great caution, if at all. Oftentimes, even in the best of hands, webs recur following surgery and can be difficult to completely resolve.

BOWED VOCAL FOLDS

The term "bowed vocal folds" is applied commonly when the vocal folds appear to be slightly concave and the glottis does not close completely (Figure 11-10). When this condition is due to muscle atrophy associated with advanced age, it can often be overcome with appropriate voice therapy. When it is due to neurological injury, such as superior laryngeal nerve paresis, the condition is more difficult to treat. Medialization procedures are reasonable in carefully selected patients with either cause (aging or paresis). Such surgery brings the vocal folds

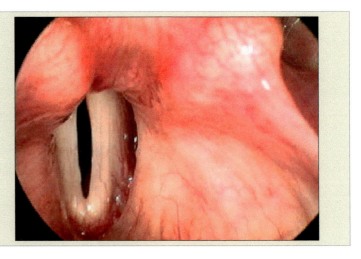

FIGURE 11–10. Bilateral vocal fold bowing.

closer together so that they can close more effortlessly, decreasing breathiness and strain during voice use.

LARYNGEAL TRAUMA

Laryngeal trauma may cause many problems in addition to the laryngeal webs discussed earlier. These include vocal fold hemorrhage, mucosal tears, laryngeal fractures, arytenoid cartilage dislocation, cricothyroid joint injury, vocal fold paralysis, and others.

When such major injuries occur in professional voice users and surgery is deemed necessary, it is advisable to involve a speech-language pathologist in the patient's care as soon as the medical condition permits, preferably prior to surgery. After surgery, the speech-language pathologist should participate in the patient's rehabilitation as soon as the patient is allowed to speak. Early involvement of the patient's singing teacher or voice coach is also helpful, so long as the teacher is known to the laryngologist, coordinates his or her plan with the laryngologist, and has proven to be knowledgeable about, and comfortable with, rehabilitation of injured voices.

PAPILLOMATOSIS

Laryngeal papillomas are wart-like growths on the vocal folds that are caused by the human papilloma virus (HPV) (Figure 11-11). Papillomas may be present at birth (congenital) or acquired later in life.

Congenital papillomas are usually acquired during birth from a mother with a history of genital warts. The exact mechanism for how infants acquire papillomas from their mothers is not completely known. In nearly all cases, the mother has a history of genital warts, which may or may not be actively present during the pregnancy or birth. Congenital papillomas can produce symptoms of hoarseness, noisy breathing, or difficulty breathing in children. The symptoms may be first apparent in early infancy, or they may not appear until mid-childhood or the adolescent years.

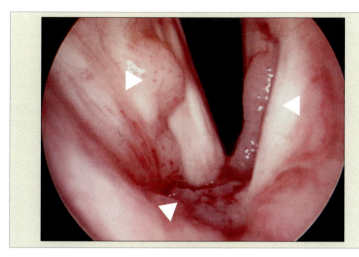

Figure 11–11. Diffuse laryngeal papilloma (*arrows*).

Acquired laryngeal papillomatosis occurs in adulthood and is acquired usually from oral sexual contact with an individual who is a carrier of the virus. Nearly 90% of the adult population in the United States has been exposed to HPV at some point in their lives, but only a small portion develop genital warts, and even a smaller portion develop laryngeal papillomas. It is unclear how the HPV vaccine will affect the incidence of new cases of laryngeal papillomas, but at the present time, the HPV vaccine is the only known way to prevent the disease. The vaccine is most effective if administered before one becomes sexually active.

Papillomas may cause hoarseness and may be associated with cancer. Patients with this condition should be followed closely in all circumstances. Symptomatic papillomas should be treated, and patients with limited areas of papilloma (especially adults with newly acquired papillomas) may be candidates for resection for possible cure or long-term control. In some cases, injection with an antiviral agent, such as cidofovir, or use of a pulsed-dye laser for resection in the office may be used instead of or in conjunction with surgery.

Because papillomas form from infection of the laryngeal tissues with the HPV virus, it is extremely difficult to eradicate completely. Usually, the goal of surgery is to remove obstructing papillomas that are limiting breathing and to remove papillomas that are causing hoarseness. Most patients require multiple procedures throughout their lifetimes to help maintain their voice and airway. It is not uncommon for a child with papillomas to have had upwards of 200 procedures by age 18 or for an adult with papillomas to need surgery as often as once every 3 months. In some patients, remission can occur for several months to several years, rendering the patient free of the need for surgery during that time period.

Precancerous and Cancerous Lesions

Control of disease must guide the treatment of vocal fold cancer, even in cases of professional voice users. However, meticulous biopsy, gently removing only suspicious tissue, usually results in satisfactory voice preservation. All cancers are graded, and a laryngologist should advise a patient of his or her "grade" of cancer. The lower grade tumors (T1 and T2) are smaller and less aggressive than the higher grades (T3 and T4).

The treatment of T1 (early stage) cancer and precancer (carcinoma in situ, also referred to as CIS or severe dysplasia) can be accomplished with either surgical resection or radiation therapy. There is some suggestion that limited surgery may produce better long-term voice results than radiation, but convincing evidence either way is lacking. For T2 cancers, radiation therapy is generally considered the treatment of choice because of the extensive surgical resection usually required to remove these tumors. In T2 tumors, radiation usually gives the better voice result.

Depending upon the presence or absence of cancer that has spread to the lymph nodes or other parts of the body, T3 and T4 cancers are usually treated with combinations of radiation therapy, chemotherapy, and/or surgical excision. Many factors are used to determine the best course of treatment in these instances, the most significant being tumor extent.

There are some long-term side effects associated with radiation, most notably a chronically dry mouth and throat, tissue swelling in the areas exposed to the radiation, and some permanent hoarseness. Short-term side effects associated with radiation and chemotherapy may occur during the course of treatment. These include mucositis (mouth sores and/or infection), weight loss, dry mouth/throat, difficulty swallowing that may require feeding tube insertion, pain with swallowing, and difficulty breathing that may require steroid treatment or tracheotomy. Close follow-up and examination with the laryngologist, oncologist (the medical doctor who administers chemotherapy), and radiation oncologist (the doctor who administers radiation therapy) during treatment will help in the early diagnosis and treatment of symptoms during chemotherapy and radiation therapy.

MISCELLANEOUS STRUCTURAL LESIONS

Other masses and structural abnormalities may occur in the larynx. These include conditions such as scar, false vocal fold cysts, epiglottic cysts, laryngoceles, and other abnormalities. These conditions usually do not affect the voice, but can in select instances. A discussion of the treatment of these lesions is beyond the scope of this book and can be found elsewhere in the literature.[1]

Which Surgical Techniques Can Be Used?

Conveniently, most vocal fold lesions (nodules, polyps, cysts, etc.) are superficial. Consequently, surgical techniques have been developed to permit the removal of lesions from the epithelium and the superficial layer of the lamina propria without disrupting the intermediate or deeper layers in most cases.

ENDOSCOPIC AND LASER TECHNIQUES

Most voice surgery is performed through the mouth after placement of an operating laryngoscope, a metal tube (endoscope), with the assistance of a microscope, a video camera, miniature surgical tools, and/or lasers. The technique is called *microscopic laryngeal surgery*. Lesions involving the vibratory margin are removed most safely using microscopic instruments such as the microscissors and microknife. Such lesions include nodules, polyps, and cysts that have not responded to voice therapy. Current techniques allow the surgeon to remove virtually nothing but the diseased tissue. Such atraumatic surgery allows healing, and good voice quality usually follows.

Although lasers are "high tech," they are not always the best choice for laryngeal surgery, at least not the lasers currently utilized. Lasers are focused heat waves concentrated into very narrow beams. The carbon dioxide (CO_2) laser and the pulsed-dye laser are the most common lasers used for laryngeal problems at the present time. The potential problem with the CO_2 laser is that a halo of laser destruction is produced surrounding the target of the laser beam. This associated heat in non-target areas may damage surrounding tissues and contribute to scar formation. Scarring that forms in response to the laser produces a segment on the vocal fold that is incapable of vibrating, and hoarseness is the result. The CO_2 laser is, however, extremely useful for selected lesions, such as cancer.

The pulsed-dye and the pulsed-KTP lasers are helpful for lesions with a rich blood supply, because they selectively vaporize red tissue, leaving the surrounding white vocal fold virtually uninjured (although in most cases some heat injury does occur to the vocal fold). The advantages of the pulsed lasers is that they can be used in the office, without the need for sedation or general anesthesia. The downside is that surgical excision is less precise than that done under the operating microscope.

When surgery is indicated for vocal fold lesions, it should be limited as strictly as possible to the area of abnormality. Virtually no place exists for "vocal cord stripping" in patients with voice problems. Even when there is a good reason to suspect malignancy, more precise surgery can and should be performed in most cases.

Precautions with Laryngeal Surgery

A detailed discussion of laryngeal surgery is beyond the scope of this publication. However, a few points are worthy of special emphasis.

Surgery for *vocal nodules* should be avoided whenever possible and should almost never be performed without an adequate trial of expert voice therapy, including patient compliance with therapeutic suggestions. In most cases, a minimum of 6 to 12 weeks of observation should be allowed while the patient is using therapeutically modified voice techniques under the supervision of a certified speech-language pathologist and possibly a singing teacher. Proper voice use rather than voice rest (silence) is correct therapy. The surgeon should not perform surgery prematurely under pressure from the patient for a "quick cure" and early return to voice performance. Permanent destruction of voice quality is a very real complication.

Because nodules are, in essence, scar tissue that has formed on the vocal folds in response to improper voice use, any surgical procedure to remove that scar will inevitably result in more scar tissue formation. Even after expert surgery, voice quality may be diminished by further scarring, and the decision to perform surgery to remove vocal fold nodules should be made only if voice therapy has had insufficient benefit and if the patient is unable to use his or her voice professionally to satisfaction with the nodules present. In this instance only, the patient should understand that removal of the nodules may improve the voice enough to allow vocal performance, but because some scar tissue is likely to form, it is unlikely to return the voice to its normal, healthy sound.

There are also other potential complications of voice surgery. Although they are uncommon or rare, they may be seen occasionally, even if the surgeon and patient do everything correctly. They include the following (among others):

1) swelling with airway obstruction requiring tracheotomy (breathing tube);
2) chipping or fracture of a tooth by the laryngoscope;
3) bleeding;
4) infection;
5) scarring resulting in permanent hoarseness;
6) recurrence of the problem (or a new mass such as a cyst or granuloma) requiring additional therapy (medications, voice therapy and/or surgery);
7) injury to the larynx, such as arytenoid dislocation;
8) tongue lacerations from the laryngoscope;
9) tongue numbness or altered taste;
10) jaw pain or discomfort from having the mouth opened widely to accommodate the laryngoscope; and
11) neck pain from having the neck extended during surgery, and others.

One of the most common factors contributing to poor healing and/or the development of scarring after surgery is *reflux* onto the fresh surgical wound. In all patients, even those with no symptoms or diagnosis of reflux, elevation of the head of bed before and for at least 6 months after surgery will help to prevent nighttime reflux that is positional. In those with a diagnosis of reflux, meticulous attention to taking the reflux medication before and after surgery is imperative.

Vocal fold contact, especially contact that results from forceful vocal fold closure, will contribute to scar formation in the early (first 3 months) post-operative period. For these reasons, many surgeons recommend a period of complete voice rest (no vocalization) and/or a period of modified voice rest (limited vocalization) after surgery.

Coughing, vomiting, and straining (such as occurs during a bowel movement associated with constipation or while lifting a heavy object) cause pressure on the vocal folds that can contribute to scar formation after surgery as well. If these occur after surgery, or if the patient has warning signs that they may occur, the laryngologist should be notified immediately so that he or she can prescribe an appropriate remedy. For similar reasons, physical exercise (including, but not limited to, aerobics, weight-lifting, running, jogging, Tae-bo, fast-paced walking, dancing, or any other activity that causes sweating), sexual intercourse, and carrying objects (including children and pets) that weigh more than 10 pounds should also be avoided immediately after surgery and during the first 6 weeks following surgery.

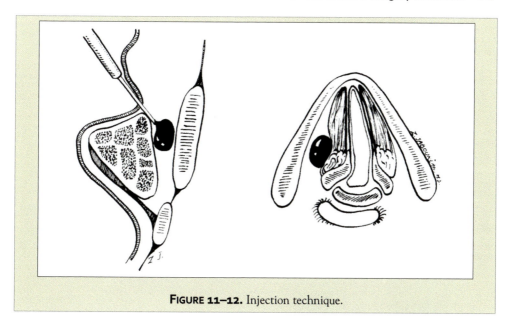

FIGURE 11–12. Injection technique.

EXTERNAL SURGICAL TECHNIQUES

New techniques of external laryngeal surgery to modify the laryngeal skeleton have become extremely useful in treating vocal fold paresis and paralysis, surgical injury, and cancer.

Until the 1980s, vocal fold paralysis was most often managed by endoscopic injection of *Teflon®* into the tissues lateral in the paralyzed vocal fold (Figure 11-12). This injection would push the paralyzed side toward the midline, allowing the normal vocal fold to meet it and thus permitting glottic closure and a better voice. Although Teflon is relatively inert, adverse reactions to it were not uncommon. Stiffness of the vocal fold from an adverse reaction to Teflon frequently impairs voice quality (Figure 11-13). Also, Teflon is hard to remove, and the voice results following such removal can be unsatisfactory and can require several surgical procedures to re-establish an acceptable voice result.

Teflon injection has been replaced by fat injection, collagen injection, injection of other materials such as fascia or hydroxylapatite, or thyroplasty.

- Thyroplasty is a technique in which a small window is cut into the thyroid cartilage, and an implant is positioned under the cartilage to push the vocal fold toward the midline; it is fairly reversible and avoids injecting a foreign body into the tissues (Figure 11-14).
- If fat injection is used, the patient's own fat is harvested from his or her abdomen and injected into the vocal fold.
- Collagen typically is purchased from a company that likewise harvests it from bodies and sterilizes it for injection.
- Fascia is the dense, collagenous tissue that covers muscles in the body; small pieces of fascia can be removed surgically from many different muscles in the body, morselized, and injected into the vocal fold.

148 *the Voice*

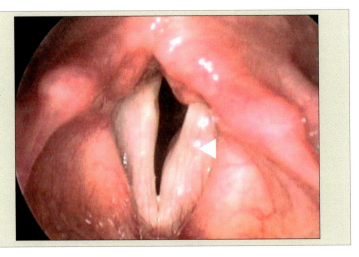

FIGURE 11–13. Left vocal fold granuloma (*arrow*), caused by a Teflon® injection, producing a convexity to the vibrating edge of the vocal fold.

- Hydroxylapatite is a synthetic material that is made from substances similar to the supporting matrix of bone. It is supplied as a paste-like material that can be injected into the larynx.

These techniques eliminate the disadvantages of Teflon, but they may pose other problems, such as resorption of the injected fat or collagen in some cases. Fat also may be used to improve vocal fold scar in selected cases.

Can Surgery Change the Pitch of a Voice?

Surgery on the laryngeal skeleton can be used to modify vocal pitch. Although such operations are done infrequently, they are valuable in certain circumstances. By closing the space between the cricoid and thyroid cartilages, the vocal folds can be lengthened and tensed, and the pitch of the voice can be raised. By cutting out vertical sections of the thyroid cartilage, the vocal folds can be shortened and their tension decreased, lowering the pitch of the voice. While these techniques are not sufficiently predictable for elective use in singers or other professional voice users, they are valuable in treating selected voice abnormalities and in altering vocal pitch in patients who have undergone gender reassignment surgery.

What Can Be Done About a Voice that Is Worse After Surgery?

Too often, the laryngologist is confronted with a desperate patient whose voice has been "ruined" by vocal fold surgery, recurrent or superior laryngeal nerve paresis or paralysis, trauma, or some other tragedy. Occasionally, the cause is as simple as a recently dislocated arytenoid that can be reduced. However, if the problem is a

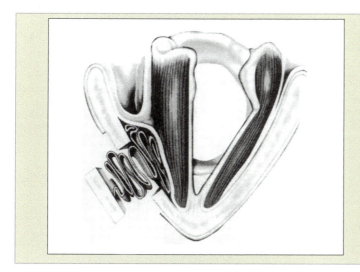

Figure 11–14. Thyroplasty technique.

vocal fold scar, decreased bulk of one vocal fold after "stripping," bowing caused by superior laryngeal nerve paralysis, or some other serious complication in a mobile vocal fold, great conservatism should be exercised. Voice therapy is nearly always helpful in optimizing compensatory strategies and minimizing fatigue, but it usually will not restore normalcy of the patient's voice. None of the available surgical procedures for these conditions is consistently effective.

If surgery is considered at all, the procedure and prognosis should be explained to the patient realistically and pessimistically. It must be understood that the chances of returning the voice to excellent quality are slim, and that it may be made worse. Steroid injection, collagen injection, and fat injection are currently the most common approaches to the treatment of vocal fold scarring. However, a great deal more research will be needed to determine the efficacy of the treatments currently available for vocal fold scarring and to establish the treatment of choice.

Summary

Patients, even professional voice users, with voice abnormalities sometimes require voice surgery. When appropriate indications are present and after appropriate preoperative care, surgery should be performed. Conditions amenable to laryngeal surgery include vocal fold nodules, cysts, polyps, hemorrhage, cancer, and others. Many of these lesions are superficial and can be treated conservatively through endoscopic laryngeal surgery. External techniques also have appropriate uses in laryngeal surgery in selected cases. Thorough preoperative evaluation, full understanding by the patient of the potential risks and outcomes involved with surgery, and the skills of an experienced and knowledgeable laryngeal microsurgeon are essential for optimal outcome, as is the consultation and support of a knowledgeable multidisciplinary voice care team.

Index

A
abdomen 20, 22-23, 23-25
abdominal surgery 24, 98-99
abuse, vocal 27-29, 61, 74, 78, 82, 89, 90, 136, 138
acetaminophen 131
acidic foods 32, 62, 114
acoustic analysis 73
acting teachers 27
acting voice specialists 37, 43-44, 48
Adam's apple 3
aerodynamic test of vocal function 71
aging, effects on voice 78-79, 124
airflow 15, 20, 72-75
alcohol 12, 31, 62, 86
allergens 61-62, 79
allergy 81-82, 130
American Academy of Otolaryngology–Head and Neck Surgery 40
American Board of Otolaryngology 38
American Bronchoesophagological Association 40
American Laryngological Association 40
American Speech-Language-Hearing Association 41
amplifier 15, 19
amplitude, vocal 17
amyloidosis 123
analgesic sprays 131
anatomy, laryngeal 1-13
androgenic hormones 62, 80
antacids 86-87, 114
antibiotics 129
antihistamines 62, 80, 82, 130
anxiety, and voice 88-89
arthritis 60
aspirin 62, 80, 83, 131
asthma 23, 62, 64, 80, 84
atrophy, vocal fold 60, 77, 80

B
back 20, 24, 100
back muscles 24
barium swallow study 112
Barrett's esophagus 105, 109
bed rest 100
Bernoulli force 16
beta-adrenergic-blocking agents 88
beta-blockers 88
beverages, for hydration 12
body posture 63, 81, 100
botulinum toxin (Botox) 69, 97, 140
breathiness 60, 65, 77, 119
breathing 20, 23, 100

C
caffeine 12, 31, 62, 114
cancer 56
cancer, laryngeal 97-98, 143
carbon dioxide (CO_2) laser 145
cartilage, laryngeal 1-13, 55, 66
   arytenoid 3, 12, 56, 107, 139
   cricoid 3
   epiglottic 3
   thyroid 3, 66
chest 20
children's voice use 78-79
chronic obstructive pulmonary disease 23, 64, 85
cold sores 78
colds 51, 82
collagen injection 147
cool-down exercises 29
corticosteroids 54, 82, 130
cortisol 65
cricoarytenoid joint 4, 60, 67, 77, 122
cricothyroid joint 142
cysts, vocal fold 18, 29, 31, 90-92, 108-110, 137-138

D
dehydration 61, 79, 82
diabetes 64, 65, 82, 124
diaphragm 20, 21-23
diet 62
direct laryngoscopy 59
diuretics 130-131
dizziness 101

E
earplugs, custom-fitted 81
edema, vocal fold 18, 52, 54, 109
edrophonium (Tensilon) 70
electromyography 56, 68
electrophysiologist 68
emphysema 23
endocrine problems 64-65, 86-87
endoscopic surgery 144
endotracheal tube, injury 55, 95
environmental irritants 61-62, 74, 79
epiglottis 3
esomeprazole (Nexium) 86
esophageal manometry 110
esophagoscopy 109, 111
esophagus 32, 103
estrogen 87
exhalation 21, 24
expiration. See exhalation
external laryngeal surgery 147
external oblique muscles 23

F
false vocal fold phonation 119
fat injection 147
fiberoptic laryngoscopy 65-67
flu 78
foods, effects on voice 32, 80
formants 20
frequency range 73
fundamental frequency 17, 19, 73

G
gargling 84
gastroesophageal reflux disease (GERD) 103, 105
gastrointestinal disorders 63, 85
glottal airflow rate 72
glottis 2
granulomas, vocal fold 108, 110, 139, 148
guaifenesin 130

H
H2-receptor antagonists 114
harmonic frequencies 19
harmonic partials 17
hearing assesment 65
hearing loss 81
heartburn 32, 63, 86, 105, 106
hemorrhage, vocal fold 18, 29, 30, 52, 54, 62, 83, 92-93, 131, 140
herbal remedies 62, 88
herpes virus infection 78
hiatal hernia 63-75, 85
hoarseness 34, 51, 55, 60-75, 77-78, 79, 119
 post-surgical 55
 prolonged 56, 79
 sudden onset 52-54
hormonal problems 64-65, 86-87
hormone replacement therapy (HRT) 87-88
human papillomavirus 56, 142
hydration 12, 31, 74, 132
hyperthyroidism 65
hypothyroidism 64

I
ibuprofen 62, 80, 83, 131
24-hour impedance testing 111
Inderal 88
infection, vocal fold 52, 82, 129
influenza 78
inhalation 20
inhalers 62, 80
internal oblique muscles 23

J
Jostle's sign 67

K
keratin 107, 109
keratosis 107, 109

L
lamina propria 5, 6, 16, 131, 135, 140
lansoprazole (Prevacid) 86
laparoscopic surgery 98
laryngeal dystonia 96-97
laryngeal electromyography 56, 68-70, 122
laryngeal evaluation 33-34, 51
laryngeal hyperfunction 18, 23, 108, 139
laryngeal papillomas 97
laryngeal surgery 23, 63, 81, 135-149
 precautions 145-147
laryngeal trauma 63, 81, 93, 142
laryngeal webs 140
laryngitis 52, 60, 62, 77, 80, 82-84
laryngitis sicca 82
laryngitis, noninfectious 82
laryngologist 27, 28, 37, 38-39, 46, 51
laryngopharyngeal reflux 103, 106, 139
 diagnosis 106-109
 symptoms 106-107
laryngoscope 107-109, 116, 144
larynx 1-13, 15, 54, 56, 103
larynx, functions 1
laser surgery 145
longevity, vocal 27-35
lower esophageal sphincter 32, 63, 86, 104, 105, 116
lubrication, vocal fold 12, 30-32, 82, 131
lung disease 85
lungs 1, 15, 17, 20, 21-23

M

maximum phonation time 72
medical history 59-75, 79
Meige's syndrome 96
menopausal vocal syndrome 88
menopause 87
menstrual problems 65
microscopic laryngeal surgery 145
microsurgery 46
milk products 32, 62, 80, 114
misuse, vocal. See abuse, vocal
MP3 players 81
mucolytics 130
multiple sclerosis 125
muscle tension dysphonia 108
muscles, abdominal 21
muscles, laryngeal 3, 4, 8, 11, 17, 23, 66, 69, 93
   cricothyroid 4, 7, 9, 66, 93
   interarytenoid 4, 10, 66
   lateral cricoarytenoid 4, 10, 66
   posterior cricoarytenoid 4, 10, 66, 125
   thyroarytenoid 4, 7, 10, 66, 125
muscular dystrophies 123
myasthenia gravis 122
myositis 123

N

nasal irrigation 84
nasopharynx 19
National Association of Teachers of Singing 43
neck trauma 54
nerve compression 124
nerve infection 124
nerve injury 10, 124
nerves, laryngeal 9, 55, 65, 78
   recurrent laryngeal 9, 55, 66, 95, 125
   superior laryngeal 9, 55, 66, 78, 93
Nissen fundoplication 116
nodules, vocal fold 18, 31, 90, 108, 136, 145
non-steroidal anti-inflammatory drugs 62, 80, 83, 131
nonsurgical treatments 129-133
nurses 37, 44-45

O

obesity 63, 85
omeprazole (Prilosec) 86
oral contraceptives 64, 86
oscillator 11, 15
otolaryngologist 37, 38, 46
oxymetazoline (Afrin) 132

P

pain, while vocalizing 61, 78
pantoprazole (Protonix) 86
papillomas, laryngeal 142
paralysis, vocal fold 11, 60, 67, 77, 93, 119
paresis, vocal fold 11, 18, 34, 54, 60, 66, 77, 78, 93, 120, 121
performance anxiety 88
Performing Arts Medicine Association 45
pH probe study, 24-hour 111
pharynx 15, 19
phonation 1, 8, 12, 18, 20, 23, 24, 29, 68, 73, 119
phoniatrist 37, 42
phonomicrosurgery 135
physical examination 65
physician assistants 45
pollution 61-62, 79
polyps, vocal fold 18, 29, 30, 91-92, 108-110, 138
post-nasal drainage 81-82
post-nasal drip 81
precancerous lesions 144
pregnancy 63, 64, 86, 99
premenstrual changes 83, 86, 130
premenstrual vocal changes 64, 86
preventative voice care 27-28, 32-33, 51-52
promotility agents 114
propranolol 88
proton-pump inhibitors 114
pulsed-dye laser 145
pulsed-KTP laser 145

R

radiation therapy, for cancer 144
rectus abdominus muscles 23
reflux 32, 34, 60, 63, 103, 146
   foods and beverages 32, 114
reflux laryngitis 32-33, 63, 78, 82, 85, 97, 103-117
   behavioral modification 112-114
   surgery 116
   treatment 112-115
reflux pillow 113
Reinke's edema 138
Reinke's space 5, 131, 138, 140
resonance 33
resonator 15, 19
respiratory problems 63, 85
respiratory system 2
ribs 22
ring (vocal) 19
robotic surgery 86

S

s/z ratio 73
scapulae 22
scar, vocal fold 89, 135
singing teacher 27, 28, 42, 135, 142
singing voice specialist 37, 42, 48

Singulair (montelukast) 130
smoke 61-62, 79, 82
smoking 23, 62, 80, 82, 97, 138
Society of Otolaryngology-Head and Neck Nurses 44
sound pressure level 73
sound waves 15, 19, 73
spasmodic dysphonia 96-97
spectral analysis 73
speech-language pathologist 27, 28, 37, 41-42, 48, 84, 132, 135, 142
spine injuries 100
spine surgery 100
spirometry 72
steam inhalation 84
strobovideolaryngoscopy 67, 137
subglottal air pressure 72
sudden change in voice 78
sulcus vocalis 140
support, breathing 20, 23-24, 32, 33, 98-99, 100
surgery, head and neck 38, 55
surgery, laryngeal 46, 135-149
swallowing 38, 103-105, 120
synkinesis 125

T
Teflon injection 147
testosterone 86
thrush infections 80, 84
thyroid gland 10
thyroid problems 64, 65, 124
thyroid surgery 10
thyroplasty 147
timbre 78
tobacco 61, 80, 114
trachea 1
transverse abdominus muscles 23

U
upper esophageal sphincter 103
upper respiratory tract infections 51, 56, 78, 82

V
vagus nerve 10
vibratory cycle 6, 17
videostroboscopy 51
vocal cord stripping 47, 145, 149
vocal emergency 46, 52, 55
vocal fatigue 60, 61-62, 65, 77, 79, 119, 120
vocal fold bowing 120, 142, 149
vocal fold disorders 89-92
vocal fold tears 18, 53, 54, 83
vocal fold trauma 18, 29, 52
vocal fold weakness 119-127
   symptoms 119
vocal folds 1, 2, 4, 5, 15, 30-32, 59-60, 66, 77
vocal function testing 71-72
vocal hygiene 27
vocal ligament 5
vocal signature 15-26
vocalis muscle 16. See thyroarytenoid
Voice and Speech Trainers Association 44
voice box 1
voice care 39
voice coaches 43-44, 142
Voice Foundation 40
Voice Handicap Index 71
voice production 1, 11, 15-26, 100
voice rest 54, 82, 84
voice scientists 37, 44, 72
voice surgery 135-149
voice surgery, timing 136
voice teacher 132
voice team 28, 37-50
voice therapy 23, 38, 42, 46, 59, 74, 89, 96-97, 126, 132-133
   preoperative 136
voice training 28, 61, 79
volume disturbance 60, 78
vomiting 52

W
warm-up exercise 29
warm-up time 63
warm-up time, prolonged 60, 78
water 12, 31

CPSIA information can be obtained
at www.ICGtesting.com
Printed in the USA
LVIC072148070513
332749LV00001B